The Penis Diet

The Penis Diet

✦

"A Comprehensive Wellness Plan for Man's Most Prized Possession"

Damon Z. Cozamanis, D.C.
Chiropractor / Author
Marc D. Grobman, D.O., F.A.C.P.
Board-Certified Internist

iUniverse, Inc.
New York Bloomington

The Penis Diet
"A Comprehensive Wellness Plan for Man's Most Prized Possession"

iUniverse books may be ordered through booksellers or by contacting:

iUniverse
1663 Liberty Drive
Bloomington, IN 47403
www.iuniverse.com
1-800-Authors (1-800-288-4677)

Because of the dynamic nature of the Internet, any Web addresses or links contained in this book may have changed since publication and may no longer be valid.

ISBN: 978-0-595-47413-4 (pbk)

ISBN: 978-0-595-91691-7 (ebk)

Printed in the United States of America

Contents

Foreword

The Penis Diet contains a very thorough review of the anatomy and physiology of erections, as well as the major causes of erectile dysfunction and impotence in men of all ages. It makes a very important message that I try to give to my patients—*the healthier you are, the healthier your erections will be.*

This book is an excellent review of positive lifestyle changes that can help improve erections, such as stress reduction, dietary factors, nutritional supplements and regular exercise. Unlike medications, these positive lifestyle changes address the actual cause of the problem and are an excellent adjunct to pharmacological management of the condition. It is clear that the treatment of erectile dysfunction not only relies on a physician's help, but the patient must also take an active role for maximum benefit.

David Cozzolino, M.D.

Acknowledgments

Marc Grobman

I would like to thank my father, Sidney, for serving as the role model for the physician I would like to be. I would like to thank my mother, Elaine, for making sure I was always dressed well, fed well and well-behaved. I would like to thank my grandparents for being strong people during the Depression years and raising my parents well so they would be good parents for me. I would like to thank my children, Alyson, Lauren and Jacob for making sure I am always awake and full of energy. Finally, I would like to thank my wife, Renee, for keeping my feet on the ground and loving me.

Damon Cozamanis

First and foremost, I would like to thank God for giving me the strength and fortitude to complete this project, and for giving me the strength, knowledge and confidence to touch the lives of others in a positive and meaningful way. I would also like to give thanks to all of those who have supported my previous endeavors and who have shown me love and support through some very rough times. You already know who you are. Last but not least, I would like to once again thank my editor Lorra Garrick, who has once again managed to help me turn a vision into a reality.

Introduction: A Solution So Simple, You Won't Believe It

Is it limp lately?

Has it been limp for a long time?

Have you tried everything and still can't get an erection? Do you feel betrayed?

How can this happen to you?

Will you ever again get a hard-on?

Don't give up. There is a way to restore virility and performance to your penis, even if it's been wilting on you for years. Never again do you have to suffer humiliation and lack of self-confidence. You can have a rock-hard sex organ by simply changing the way you take care of your body. Who would have ever thought? Yes: Change the way you treat your temple. But this isn't all about expensive drugs with side effects. It's not about magic creams or scary-looking gadgets. The solution is so simple, you won't believe it.

This book will show you the secrets to achieving and maintaining rock-hard erections that you and your lover can be proud of. *The Penis Diet* is not only for men with erectile dysfunction, but for men of all ages who want to improve their sexual performance. There will be no hassling with creams, ointments, strange devices or pills. In most cases, *The Penis Diet* offers a 100% natural solution to erectile dysfunction (ED).

When you hear "diet," what do you think of? Going hungry? Eliminating food groups? Not here. *The Penis Diet* is not a diet per se, but more of a comprehensive wellness program for one of man's most prized possessions. Contrary to what the title of this book might imply, you will not be required to consume platters of mammalian penis on this program! Whether your goal is to keep "Mr. Happy" happy, or to awaken "Mr. Sleepy," *The Penis Diet* will help you achieve your goals.

The Penis Diet incorporates the latest findings in the fields of diet and nutrition, exercise and nutritional supplementation into a cutting-edge program that will help optimize sexual function and performance in men of all ages.

In this book, we are going to:

- Describe problems with the penis and how to keep it healthy

- Delve into erectile dysfunction, its origins and how to treat it

- Discuss the anatomy, blood supply, nerve supply, physiology and overall health of this small (or large), yet powerful organ

- Review many of the obstacles to proper penis health in terms of current diseases, and then we will turn our "heads" to proper lifestyles, nutrition and medication (complementary, alternative and prescription) that can reverse disease states and return proper function to this beloved organ.

Facts About Erectile Dysfunction

Embarrassing as it may be, erectile dysfunction is a common condition.

- An estimated 10–20 million men in the U.S. suffer from this disastrous problem.

- Most men experience ED at one time or another in their lifetime.

- Studies suggest that as many as 52% of men between the ages of 40 and 70 may experience ED.

- A national health survey revealed that ED affects nearly one out of every five men over the age of 20.

ED can vary in severity, from an inability to achieve and maintain an erection (either physically or mentally), to an inability to achieve an orgasm, even though a healthy sexual desire exists. Failure to achieve an erection less than 20% of the time is not unusual, and treatment is rarely needed. Failure to achieve an erection more than 50% of the time, however, generally indicates there is a problem requiring treatment.

Because of the sensitive nature of this disorder, it often goes unreported. Women will discuss all sorts of personal body problems among themselves. You can just imagine it: a group of ladies sitting around in the powder room or kitchen, sipping tea or eating yogurt or consoling themselves with cake and ice cream while one by one, they announce their deepest, darkest secrets about their bodies.

But men? Ten men with erectile dysfunction can be in the same room for five hours, swigging beers, munching on pretzels and eating hotdogs, and *never* will the topic of ED "come up." You can be sure of that. They'll be chatting all night long about their cars and favorite movie stars while they hide how much of a nervous wreck they've been because their penis can't get harder than a deflated balloon when in the company of even the hottest women.

This should not be something to withhold from your physician because, as we will discuss later on, a problem with erections often heralds disease in other areas of the body. To ignore this difficulty means we lose an opportunity to treat a condition when it is just beginning, thus making it harder more difficult to regain health. As "hard" as it is to discuss, it is a subject that could save your life (and we are not just speaking about your social life here).

1

How the Penis Works

Anatomy of the Penis

The penis is like the space shuttle's rocket booster (talk about a phallic symbol!) with a covering, of course. Inside the penis are two cylinders, called the corpus cavernosa. These are filled with a spongy tissue rich in blood supply, fibrous tissues and smooth muscle. The corpus cavernosa are covered by a soft membrane, or wrap. The urethra is a tube that basically runs from the bladder through the prostate into the underside of the penis, to allow for emptying of the bladder during urination. Into this tube empties the seminal vesicles, which carry sperm from the testicles during ejaculation, which allows for passage of sperm out of the body.

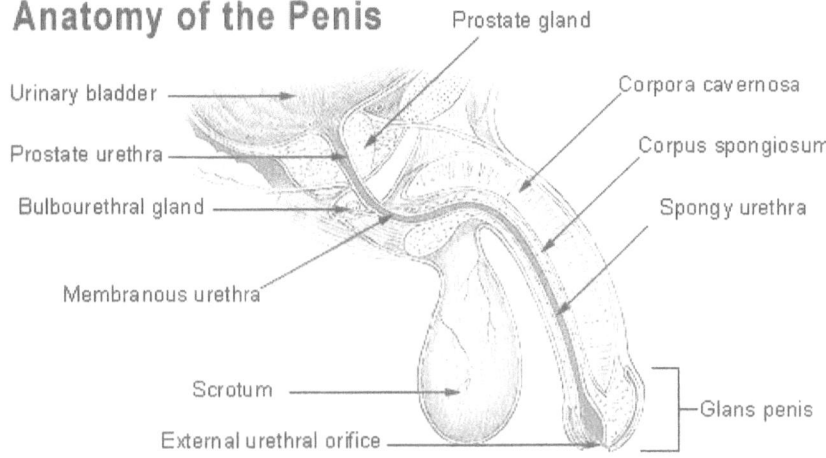

Anatomy of the Penis

Prostate gland

Urinary bladder

Corpora cavernosa

Prostate urethra

Corpus spongiosum

Bulbourethral gland

Spongy urethra

Membranous urethra

Scrotum

Glans penis

External urethral orifice

How An Erection Occurs

As simple as it may seem, achieving an erection is a complex process. It involves psychological impulses from the brain, adequate levels of the male sex hormone testosterone, a properly functioning nervous system, and sufficient blood supply to the penis.

When we are sexually stimulated, electrical signals from the brain cause the nerves in the penis to release nitric oxide. Nitric oxide is synthesized from the amino acid L-arginine. Nitric oxide increases the production of c-GMP in the corpus cavernosa (see diagram above). c-GMP causes the corpus cavernosa to relax and fill with blood, which causes the penis to expand, leading to an erection.

Connective tissue traps the blood in the penis and keeps the erection firm. If there is something interfering with any or all of these conditions, a full erection will not occur, leading to ED. After climax, or an unexpected interruption (the parents are home!) the smooth muscles in the penis contract and cause the trapped blood to empty. The penis then softens like a balloon that has just lost all its air.

As complex as this all seems, let's just say that nitric oxide is a key that opens the door for blood to flow into the penis. If you have enough of it and it is of good quality, then all is well. Any disease that can interfere with the quality or quantity of nitric oxide (or blood flow into the penis) can upset the apple cart. As you can guess, the more complicated a system is, the easier it is to disrupt. Now we can begin to review the ways that erections can be prevented, interrupted or deflated. Just remember the two key items here:

1. nitric oxide, and

2. blood flow into the penis.

2

The Many Causes of Erectile Dysfunction

Causes of Erectile Dysfunction

Aging is a primary cause of ED, but this condition happens to a lot of middle-aged and even younger men. Don't let those Bob Dole commercials fool you. It's just that senior citizens are less likely to be embarrassed about discussing it with their doctors because they can always use age as an excuse.

Psychological Causes of ED

Stress can really do a bad number on your penis. If yours has been wilting lately, ask yourself some questions. Have you been experiencing financial problems or turbulence on the job? Any anxiety in your life? In-law problems? Can't stand your boss at work? Neighbor's dog keeps pooping in your yard? Depression? Excessive guilt? How about low self-esteem or marital issues? ED from the wear-and-tear of mental issues, or stress, most often strikes younger men. Remember: Stress, anxiety and depression lead the pack of psychological factors that can make a penis just give up and droop.

How does mental angst make a penis not work? High stress levels cause fatigue and stunt sex drive as a result of increased cortisol levels. You've heard of cortisol, right? This is the "stress toxin" that's been linked to excess fat in the belly. But it does more than that. Surging cortisol can throw off metabolism, energy levels and obstruct libido. You'll have difficulty relaxing. Feeling uptight and wound-up, with your body's systems out of synch, it's no wonder that your penis will eventually pay the price for this.

This needs to happen only once in order for a man to develop a lot of fear that it will happen a second time. This fear will compound things and lead to performance anxiety, or a fear of sexual failure. He ends up becoming locked in a groove from which there is no way out. He anticipates erectile failure so much that it's all he can think about when he's with a woman, and his prophecy of failure then becomes true. Sometimes, men in this predicament will take drugs to treat depression, not knowing that side effects from "medications" can even cause or aggravate ED!

Physical Causes of ED

The physical causes of ED are related to a breakdown or damage to the sequence of events that lead to an erection. In a study published in the February 2007 issue of *The American Journal of Medicine*, researchers reported that erectile dysfunction was significantly and independently associated with age, cardiovascular disease, diabetes and lack of physical activity. There was an especially high prevalence of erectile dysfunction among men with diabetes and high blood pressure. The associations between erectile dysfunction and diabetes, and other known cardiovascular risk factors, should serve as powerful motivators for male patients for whom diet and lifestyle changes are needed to improve their cardiovascular risk profile.

Diabetes

Diabetes is what physicians call a small-vessel disease. Diabetes can cause nerve and artery damage that can make achieving an erection difficult. Between 35% and 50% of men with diabetes experience ED, and this risk increases with age, according to the National Institutes of Health.

In uncontrolled diabetes, the same processes that cause damage in other parts of the body also damage the vessels and nerves leading to the penis. As the blood sugar rises over time, it "poisons" the small blood vessels of the penis. As the tiny blood vessels become diseased, they clog with plaque, narrow, and blood flow is disrupted, leading to ED. If you have diabetes, keeping your blood sugar in a healthy range will help prevent the damage in the body that leads to ED. By maintaining a healthy diet, getting regular exercise, and taking the appropriate medicine, men with diabetes may be able to avoid diabetes-related ED.

Hypertension (High Blood Pressure)

Hypertension is often accompanied by obesity, smoking, high cholesterol, poor exercise and diabetes—all of which can damage penile blood vessels and increase the risk for ED. Individuals who suffer from hypertension have also been found to exhibit low nitric oxide production.

If you have high blood pressure, it is very important that you follow your doctor's advice. Take your blood pressure medication as prescribed, and keep your blood pressure in a healthy range. Also, keep in mind that if you are overweight, losing weight can reduce your blood pressure. Losing just 5% or 10% of your current body weight can be an effective way to control high blood pressure.

Another way to lower blood pressure is to exercise; a 30-minute nonstop, brisk walk, done daily, should lower blood pressure. If you're already exercising, then either increase intensity (but make sure you don't go overboard, since rigorous weight routines will increase blood pressure during the actual routines; always consult with your doctor on this). On the other hand, you can still increase intensity without being too strenuous, especially if your current routine lacks fire. For example, if all you've been doing for cardio is walking, maybe it's time to start jogging or take a cardio kickboxing class to make sure you're getting a good workout every day.

Adding potassium-rich foods and supplements to your diet and avoiding salt can also help reduce blood pressure. Increasing your intake of bananas or fresh broccoli can help to assure a proper potassium-sodium balance. Be sure to speak with your doctor if you plan to take potassium supplements. Too much potassium in your bloodstream can be dangerous.

Vascular Disease

Vascular diseases are those that affect the blood vessels. These maladies include atherosclerosis (hardening of the arteries), hypertension and high cholesterol. These medical conditions, which account for 70% of physically-related causes of ED, all restrict blood flow to the heart, the brain and, in the case of ED, the penis.

Elevated cholesterol, over time, lines the arteries with plaque. This is a sneaky process that occurs silently and leads to diminution of life-sustaining and penis-filling blood. In the worst case scenario, a stable lining of plaque can fracture or break and send a tiny clot to the brain, causing a stroke; or the clot can make its way to the heart and cause a heart attack; or, perish the thought, to Mr. Happy, causing a penile infarct (though this is exceptionally rare, if ever, seen).

Erectile dysfunction is now being proven to be, if not a risk factor, then a marker for coronary artery disease. Let's face it: Once the blood supply to the penis has been hampered, the heart is not going to be far behind. As physicians, we are now being urged to ask all men over 40 years of age with ED to have a stress test to look for premature heart disease—as if not being able to have sex weren't bad enough! By maintaining healthy eating habits, sticking to consistent exercise, and taking the appropriate medicine, men can lower their cholesterol and reduce their risk of ED and heart disease.

Overweight and Obesity

Leading a sedentary lifestyle is associated with being overweight. Being overweight increases the risk of diabetes, high blood pressure and vascular disease, all of which can reduce blood flow to the penis and ultimately lead to ED. As you will soon learn, adhering to a regular exercise regimen, combined with a healthy eating pattern, can greatly reduce the risk of ED and improve sexual function.

Neurological (Nerve and Brain) Diseases

The nervous system plays a vital part in achieving and maintaining an erection, and it is common for men with diseases afflictions such as stroke, multiple sclerosis (MS), Alzheimer's disease, and Parkinson's disease to experience ED. This is due to an interruption in the transmission of nerve impulses between the brain and the penis.

The physical causes of ED are not only disease-related. There are many other potential causes, including surgery to treat diseases such as prostate and bladder cancer (which can traumatize nerves in that area), injury to the spinal cord, imbalances of hormones such as thyroid hormones, prolactin and testosterone, and even medication.

Hormones

Hormonal illnesses are also an important player in this game. Testosterone is thought of as being more involved in libido, but if there is a deficiency, then a full and firm erection will be lacking. Decreased thyroid hormone production will produce a body and person who lacks energy, gains weight, becomes constipated and lethargic, and will suffer from an absence of any interest in "playful" activity.

Increased prolactin, a hormone secreted by the hypothalamus in the brain, can produce erectile dysfunction by decreasing the secretion of gonadotropin-releasing hormone (GnRH), and thus also depress testosterone production. Depression, anxiety, bipolar disorder, and neuroses also can interfere with your penis' proper function. More examples of psychogenically produced ED are performance anxiety, conflict over sexual preferences (male and female gender, not position), fear of pregnancy or STDs, and prior sexual abuse. All of this means the picture is not a simple one, and again we urge you to discuss this malady with your physician.

Medication (including over-the-counter)

While physicians use medication to treat illnesses, many times side effects do appear and can affect Mr. Happy. There are over 200 types of prescription drugs that may cause ED. If you are having penis problems, take a look at your medicine cabinet. Even over-the-counter drugs can cause a limp, sagging, uncooperative penis. While these medications may treat a disease or condition, in doing so they can affect a man's hormones, nerves, or blood circulation, resulting in ED, or increasing the risk of ED.

Medications that can produce ED are:

- diuretics

- blood pressure medication

- drugs to prevent or treat heart conditions

- antidepressants and tranquilizers

- allergy medications

- hormones

- chemotherapy agents

- anticholinergics

- recreational drugs such as cocaine, marijuana and alcohol (leading to "Whiskey Dick").

Lifestyle Factors

The "fun" way of living can actually cause problems with your penis. Drinking, smoking and eating your favorite junk foods can make a penis wilt. So can lounging around too much or using illegal drugs. Is that joint worth a withered penis? Men can take active steps to prevent ED or improve their condition by adopting a healthier lifestyle.

Smoking

Smoking increases a person's risk of atherosclerosis (hardening of the arteries), which can reduce blood flow throughout the body, including to the penis, impairing a man's ability to gain an erection. Quitting smoking can help some men partly or fully restore erectile function.

There's no way around it: Men who smoke have an increased incidence of ED. A study of 4,462 Vietnam War veterans showed that smoking increases the risk of ED by around 50% for men in their 30s and 40s. Other damage caused by smoking to male sexual health includes reduced volume of ejaculate, lowered sperm count, abnormal sperm shape and impaired sperm mobility (shooting blanks). And to think that at one time, smoking was glamorized by Hollywood filmmakers as a sign of male virility!

Excessive Drinking

More than two drinks a day can inhibit erectile functioning by causing a restriction in blood flow to the penis, and can impede the production of testosterone, negatively affecting sex drive and erections. A glass or two of alcohol can help decrease inhibitions, but excessive intake often impairs performance.

Illegal Drug Use

Marijuana, cocaine, and other illegal drugs can cause impotence by damaging blood vessels and/or restricting blood flow to the penis.

Unhealthy Diet

Diets high in saturated fat (burgers, hot dogs, pizza, pastries) and sugar (soda, candy, pastries, ice cream) increase the risk for obesity, diabetes, hypertension and vascular disease, all of which can lead to ED.

The last word here should be that often, there is not just one cause of ED. Usually it is a constellation of problems from many areas that are the culprits. Our next section will deal with how to find the best treatment for Mr. Happy.

3

The Medical Workup for ED

I am reminded of the 20-year-old male who made an emergency appointment with me because he could no longer have 4–5 erections each night with his girl-friend, as he had done at age 18! He was actually upset he lost the erection after each climax. After reviewing the way things are supposed to happen, he left with a better understanding of the process, if not a better performance.

There are many tests that can diagnose the causes of ED. We will review them all. Your family physician should first perform a thorough history and physical to assess your general health. Medications should be reviewed along with past medical and surgical history. Findings like an abnormal pattern of hair growth or breast enlargement can indicate certain hormonal problems, whereas poor pulses or high blood pressure can hint at cardiovascular troubles.

A general review and discussion of your concerns and problems are often the best first steps. Understanding the process often leads to the correction of certain habits that are damaging to your health. It can also lead to reasonable expectations of what can really be achieved.

Blood Work

Blood work should include an assay, or determination of the amount of certain hormones present in the blood stream. The basic labs should include:

- a blood sugar test

- white and red cell count

- kidney function (BUN and creatinine)

- liver function tests for hepatitis

- PSA (prostate-specific antigen) for prostate cancer and benign prostatic hypertrophy

- FSH, LH and testosterone (the sex hormones) test.

Your physician should ask if you awaken from sleep at any time with an erection. This can be an embarrassing question to ask *and* to answer. It is normal for a male to have 4–5 erections each night during sleep. Some of us never realize we have had erections during sleep. Men unable to achieve an erection due to a mental issue will still have erections during sleep. The ability to do so indicates that the system works, but just not at the desired moments, which demands a specific workup.

If you cannot be certain whether erections occur while you sleep, the nocturnal penile tumescence (NPT) test is indicated. Most men have 3 to 5 full erections while sleeping. The NPT test is used to help determine if a man is having normal erections during sleep.

A simple ring-like device containing plastic films is placed around the penis before going to bed at night. If an erection occurs, the plastic film will expand and break. There are also electronic versions of this test which provide details as to the number, duration and stiffness of the erection.

Hormone Tests

Your family physician or urologist can do the next round of tests. These include follicle-stimulating hormone (FSH), luteinizing hormone (LH), thyroid-stimulating hormone (TSH), prolactin and testosterone (total and free concentrations). These hormones are produced in the pituitary gland, a tiny gland centrally located under the brain.

If one hormone is overproduced, that area of the brain can grow, squeezing out the others, thus leading to deficiencies. If testing reveals an overabundance of one or more of these hormones, an MRI is next ordered to assess the size of the hypothalamus. Many times medication can be used to reverse the problem, but in some cases a neurosurgeon may need to remove the overgrown area, called a macroadenoma.

Penis Ultrasound

The next group of tests would make the Marquis de Sade proud and jealous. An ultrasound of the penis is probably the next test to order. This would be to determine if there are leaks in the vascular system, signs of clogged arteries, scarring or calcification of the erectile tissues.

A hormone, prostaglandin, is injected into the penis tissue. This causes the erection to occur artificially, and then the ultrasound is used to measure the penile blood pressure and compare it to the flaccid state. This is probably the most comfortable of the tests to review.

Nerve Function

The next test is for penile nerve function. The testing physician pinches the head of the penis, which should immediately cause the anus to contract if nerve function is indeed normal. Who wouldn't want this test done?

Testing for Stiffness

The NPT test (nocturnal penile tumescence testing) measures the actual stiffness of the penis during nocturnal erections, if they do occur. Unfortunately, they can only measure one erection. If more occur, we could not say how many and how strong they are. The point here would be that erections DO occur and they are strong enough to be measured, so other avenues of diagnosis can be pursued.

Penile biothesiometry can assess the sensitivity of the penile nerve system along the glans (head) and shaft of the penis. Any decrease in awareness of the vibrations point to damage in the pelvic area.

Pressure Testing

Penile cavernosometrics reveal pressure within the corpora cavernosa after injecting prostaglandin (our old friend from above), followed by saltwater. The volume of saltwater (saline) needed to maintain the erection is the key. Dye can then be injected if the volume keeps changing, to discover any leaks in the venous system. The dye is held in place by a tourniquet at the base of the shaft. Wow, what a picture! Dye studies may also be done for the arterial system after pelvic trauma. Just thinking of these tests makes us sweat.

"For more information about mechanical means to increase penis girth or length, see page 75."

4

"How Can I Prevent Erectile Dysfunction?"

Preventing Erectile Dysfunction

For people who are at risk for developing ED (all men), taking active steps to prevent its occurrence will not only help you maintain erectile function, but will also help you lead a healthier life overall. Some steps you can take to prevent ED include:

- Stop smoking. It just isn't cool. This includes cigars and pipes. If you lack the willpower, then remind yourself, "I'm quitting for my penis."

- Exercise regularly. This doesn't mean you got in your daily exercise quota because you helped your wife or girlfriend load the dishwasher. When we say exercise, we mean exercise—as in jogging or rigorous walking, weight workouts, lap swimming, hiking or a sweaty game of racquetball.

- Follow a healthy diet. This doesn't just mean portion control, but avoidance or restriction of harmful ingredients like sugar, trans fats, hydrogenated oils and heavily processed foods.

- Maintain a healthy weight. Have you always skirted this issue and instead convinced yourself that you are "big boned" or "large framed"? Many tall men do this. Being extra tall is no excuse for carrying around extra fat. Have a personal trainer give you a body fat test with skin-fold calipers if you think your extra girth is simply from "big bones."

- Review your medications with your doctor and ask about possible substitutions for those that may cause ED. Write down notes and questions for your physician; you may as well get as much out of the visit as possible, considering how much it costs to spend just 15 minutes in a doctor's office.

- Avoid excessive alcohol. Go straight to the gym after work instead of the bar.

- Avoid illegal drugs. Yes, it's that simple: Avoid them.

- If you have a chronic illness such as high blood pressure, diabetes or kidney disease, follow your doctor's guidelines to keep these conditions under control.

5

Medical Treatments for Erectile Dysfunction

Treatment of Erectile Dysfunction

Over the centuries, therapy for erectile dysfunction has included powder from the horn of a unicorn to magical creams and ointments to prescription drugs. If you currently suffer from ED, you have the option of utilizing a variety of medical treatments, natural alternatives, or a combination of the two.

In this section we will review the treatments from proven to not-so-proven, tried-and-true to please-oh-please. Remember, this is not an illness without a cause. Remedies should be directed at the root of the problem; therefore, it is critical to have the above diagnostics performed.

Medical Options

Hormonal Replacement

If a hormonal deficiency is found, replenishing that hormone is key. Testosterone is available in four basic forms and can be injected into the buttocks every two weeks at a dose of 100–200 mg. This dose should be enough to restore NOR-MAL levels, which in turn should restore libido, decrease fat, increase lean muscle mass and increase physical and mental energy.

If you don't like getting shot in the butt every two weeks, there are two other forms of replacement, including a gel and a patch. Most insurance companies variably pay for the patch and gel, and coverage can actually vary from year to year, so work with your physician to investigate your options. Testosterone replacement can help restore your sex drive, but may not cheer up Mr. Happy enough for penetration. Additional treatments may also be required.

Drawbacks: A potential downside is injection site infection or pain, and this treatment should not be used in men with prostate cancer.

Vacuum Constriction Devices—Penis Pumps

If there is a blood delivery problem, there are a number of devices that have been used over the last 20–30 years to overcome this. Vacuum constriction devices (have you seen "Austin Powers"?) have been employed to draw blood into the penis, and then a ring is used at the base of the penis shaft to contain the blood during sexual activity. This device can be quite awkward and may interfere with the ambience of the moment.

Drawbacks: Contrary to popular belief, these devices will not increase the size of Mr. Happy. They should not be used in men with sickle-cell disease or those on anticoagulants, for fear of bleeding or blood clots. If you draw your partner into the process, though, the teamwork aspect could be quite effective.

Intraurethral Medication

Speaking about teamwork, here is a perfect remedy: intraurethral medication. That's right: One takes a tiny straw with a pill in it, places it into the urethra and deposits the pill about a centimeter down. Then the pill must be absorbed, so the hands are put to work, rolling the shaft back and forth, allowing for dispersal of medication and stimulation of the penis.

Drawbacks: This technique can produce irritation of the urethra, which can make Mr. Happy a bit uncomfortable. It is effective in about 65% of cases.

Penile Injections with Vasoactive Drugs

If all else fails, an injection of a prostaglandin-like substance directly into the corpus cavernosa, at the base of the penis shaft, may be your best bet. Vasoactive drugs help increase blood flow into the penis. Before you get your shorts in a bunch, there are not a lot of nerve fibers at the base of the shaft, so it should not be that uncomfortable—"should" being the important word. The effects can last 1–2 hours. The success rate is 95%.

Drawbacks: There is an auto-injector if you are faint of heart or find it too difficult to inject on your own. This is not a proper form of therapy for men with blood clot problems or sickle-cell disease, and can lead to liver damage, and rarely, lead to a never-ending erection. As you can imagine, this form of cure has a high discontinuation rate. Ohh, the lengths we will go to for Mr. Happy.

Surgery—Penile Implants

In rare instances, to correct leaks of the blood vessels we spoke of previously, surgery may be needed. You will also need surgery for the implantation of a semirigid rod or inflatable device to produce an erection.

Drawbacks: A urologist with specialized training should perform this particular operation, because complications like device malfunction and infection are possible, and the cost is high.

Oral Medications

Oral medications are the easiest options today. Newer drugs brought to the market in the last eight years have revolutionized the treatment for this condition and have brought much joy to men and the pharmaceutical industry. These medications work by blocking the chemical c-GMP that we discussed previously. This leads to an increase in nitric oxide, which will relax the smooth muscles of the penis to encourage blood flow into the corpus cavernosa, producing a very gleeful and proud Mr. Happy.

This option has a 75–80% success rate in all men with ED, in most men with psychological causes, and in 40% of those having had radical prostate surgery for cancer. The effects can last 4–36 hours, depending on which preparation you use.

Drawbacks: These pills can be quite expensive, at $6–12 per pill, and coverage is even more variable among insurance companies. Experimentation may be necessary, because one of these medications will not work for all men.

Psychotherapy

We should not avoid discussing psychotherapy. Mental illness is a significant burden in this country. Those who have it and those who have yet to be diagnosed are weighed down and always living under a dark cloud that interferes with every aspect of their lives. It slows them down, robs them of any joy, and depletes their energy to do anything. Counseling can be very effective, along with medication.

Some of you may not be ready or willing to accept the "warm and fuzzy" approach with psychotherapy. You may believe you can "tough it out" on your own. There are those of you who may not even realize there is a problem! Whomever you are, your physician should be able to diagnose your condition, or at least refer you to someone who can.

Psychotherapy can define the root of the problem and get you to confront it head-on and manage it. On the other hand, without medication, you may not be able to muster the courage or willpower to deal with your issues, so do not rule this out without a discussion with your physician.

Medications like serotonin-uptake inhibitors (SSRI), dopamine-uptake inhibitors, atypical psychotropics, and norepinephrine-uptake inhibitors (SNRI) all have wonderful success rates with few side effects: Some of the SSRI's can reduce libido, while an SNRI may delay orgasm (not necessarily a problem).

6

Natural "Cures" for Erectile Dysfunction.

The Natural Approach

One of the best ways to achieve permanent elimination of erectile dysfunction is to change the way you live. A new study appearing in the *American Journal of Medicine (2007)* now confirms this. The study revealed that nearly 1 in 5 men experience ED, but that simple lifestyle changes may be all it takes to ward off the problem.

Researchers examined the prevalence of ED and its association with other health problems in a sample of more than 2,100 men, age 20 and older. The study showed that men with heart disease risk factors, diabetes, or a sedentary lifestyle were much more likely to report ED than healthier, more physically active men.

The study's results showed that:

• Almost 90% of men with ED had at least one risk factor for heart disease, such as high blood pressure, elevated cholesterol, smoking, or diabetes.

• Fifty percent of men with diabetes reported ED.

• Men with diabetes were three times more likely to have ED than men without diabetes, even after adjusting for other risk factors.

• Men who were sedentary, such as those who hadn't engaged in vigorous physical activity for at least a month, were much more likely to have ED than men who were physically active.

The findings of this study are consistent with previous studies, and suggest that making simple lifestyle changes may be all it takes to stave off the onset of ED. The good news is that these simple changes target the direct cause of the problem, rather than merely treating the symptoms of the problem, as medications do. Now we will learn a little more about *The Penis Diet.*

The Penis Diet is more than a diet. It is a complete wellness program for your penis (and body). The program includes:

- proper diet and nutrition

- exercise recommendations

- stress reduction techniques

- a very specific nutritional supplementation program aimed at attacking both the causes and symptoms of ED

The lifestyle modifications discussed in this program are designed to work together in a synergistic fashion, meaning the total response or effect is greater than the sum of the parts. In other words, healthy eating and regular workouts are beneficial, independent of one another, but when they are done simultaneously, the benefit is even greater.

If you want to achieve the maximum benefit rewards from the program, you need to be committed in all areas—not just the ones you find enjoyable. In other words, let's say that you're may be a real animal in the gym, but if your diet is full of junk, you'll be missing the boat. Conversely, your diet may be as pure as a stream in the Alps, but if you don't exercise or learn how to manage the stress in your life, Mr. Happy will be Mr. Floppy.

You also need to make a full-time commitment to the program. Eating a few salads here and there and taking a short walk a few days a week will not counteract a diet heavy in fried and sugary foods and a sedentary lifestyle. If you expect your penis to work full-time, then so should you. It's that simple.

Program guidelines are as follows:

- If you smoke—QUIT!

- Manage STRESS.

- EXERCISE more.

- Adopt a penis-friendly DIET.

- Drink more WATER.

- Use NUTRITIONAL SUPPLEMENTS wisely.

- Have more SEX.

- Consult your DOCTOR.

Smoking Kills You and Your Penis

Research suggests that men who smoke a pack or more of cigarettes daily are nearly 50% more likely to have erectile dysfunction compared with nonsmokers. Men who smoke one pack or less a day are about 25% more likely to report difficulties maintaining an erection. Smoking kills erections! Puffing away accelerates hardening and narrowing of the arteries. It just stands to reason that what harms blood vessels in one area of the body, harms them in other areas. When arteries become hard and narrowed, blood flow is reduced. Hard arteries = a soft penis.

Yes, indeed, this amounts to a "Mr. Softy." Quitting smoking can help some men partly or fully restore erectile function. If you currently smoke, we recommend dropping this deadly, stinking habit immediately, which is a real turnoff to many women anyway.

Smoking does nothing to improve your sex appeal or sexuality. Your breath will stink like an ashtray, your teeth will become yellow, grey or brown, your skin will wrinkle prematurely, and you'll likely be unable to achieve a strong enough erection to satisfy your lover—if she already hasn't rejected you because of your tobacco breath and stained teeth. Smoking also snuffs out your stamina and will result in a lackluster performance in the bedroom, even if you do not suffer from ED. Hanging out in smoke-filled restaurants and bars on a regular basis can also lead to ED.

Is Your Penis Stressed Out?

Stress is a serious health problem, and according to medical researchers, 75–90% of all visits to primary care physicians are for complaints and conditions that are, in some way, stress-related. Every week, over 115 million people take some form of medication for stress-related symptoms.

Ongoing stress may result in ED, which in turn increases stress. The emotional impact the condition can have on a man and his partner can be just as difficult. It is common for men with ED to feel anger, frustration, sadness, or a lack of confidence, all of which can affect a man's libido or performance. We're talking about a vicious cycle here.

Top Ten Stressors

1. Death of spouse

2. Divorce

3. Marital separation

4. Jail term

5. Death of close family member

6. Personal injury or illness

7. Marriage

8. Fired at work

9. Marital reconciliation

10. Retirement

Our bodies are designed to feel stress and react to it. It keeps us alert and ready to avoid danger. But it is not always possible to avoid or change events that may cause stress, and it is easy to feel trapped and unable to cope.

An example of how we're supposed to deal with stress can be visualized with how ancient man lived. He counteracted stress the moment it occurred, because the opportunity was there: For example, if he spotted a snake, he was able to instantly react by leaping onto some boulders and running away from it (or clubbing it with a tree branch). This was the kind of stress that early man encountered: survival stress. And his physical reaction to it counteracted the hormonal response to the stress.

But when hormones that are released as a result of stress are not counteracted with intense physical activity or avoidance of the stress agent, this accumulation of stress hormones can compromise health, leading to inefficient penile functioning, i.e., a "soft-on." Modern man typically becomes stressed during times that he simply cannot counteract the stress with intense physical activity. A classic example is being chewed out by his boss at work. Feeling his blood boiling, he goes to his cubicle, sits and fumes. Another classic example is sitting trapped in a car, in a hurry, but stuck in a traffic jam. The mounting stress can be unbearable, yet all the body can do is remain totally inert.

When stress persists, the body begins to break down, and illnesses can flourish. An erection is a complex process that involves both physical and psychological components. Chronic stress can interfere with the psychological component of an erection and make it difficult, if not impossible, to achieve or maintain an erection.

Chronic exposure to stress can also increase the levels of stress hormones in the body, especially cortisol. High levels of cortisol have also been linked to weight gain, digestive disorders, sleep disturbances and loss of sex drive. Other stress hormones trigger the release of fats into the bloodstream that increase cholesterol levels and may accelerate the buildup of fatty plaques within the arteries.

To successfully combat the effects of stress, you must first identify its primary sources. Truly make an attempt to eliminate or reduce your exposure to stressors. Unfortunately, this is easier said than done if the stressor is your boss at work. You'd love to take a punch at the buffoon, but if you do, you'll get fired, and you have the mortgage to pay and three mouths at home to feed. Talk about stress!

But being trapped in a crummy work environment doesn't mean your only options are to engage in negative coping patterns such as smoking, drinking and overeating. If you already are succumbing to these crippling habits, they must also be replaced with more constructive measures such as relaxation techniques (meditation and deep breathing), vigorous exercise, stretching routines, listening to soothing music, and holistic supplementation.

The mirror image of the "stress" response is the "relaxation response," identified by Dr. Herbert Benson in 1974. The relaxation response appears to be an antidote to the effects of the stress reaction. The key to activating this response lies in the stimulation of the parasympathetic nervous system. When this system is stimulated through a rhythmical activity such as deep breathing patterns or meditation, the individual will begin to experience a sense of calm and relaxation, leading to a reduction in blood pressure, perspiration, muscle tension and breathing rate, plus increased relaxation.

Practicing techniques that elicit the relaxation response have been found to enhance the effectiveness of the body's natural defenses and self-repair mechanisms. Other positive changes associated with the relaxation response include improved emotional well-being and better coping skills when encountered with nerve-jarring situations.

A variety of techniques can be used to elicit the relaxation response, most of which are the basis of mind/body medicine. Two of the most common and effective techniques used to elicit this response include deep breathing exercises and meditation. Best of all, these techniques take just a few minutes a day and can be practiced in the comfort of your home or office.

Deep Breathing

Under stressful situations, our breathing patterns become more rapid and shallow, the heart rate increases and the muscles in the body become tense. When most adults breathe, they tend to fill only their upper chest with air, a sign of shallow breathing. Chest breathing is similar to the type of breathing induced during the "fight or flight" stress response.

Over time, the body can create the edgy feelings associated with that response. Deep breathing slows the heart rate, dilates blood vessels and relaxes muscles. It is also thought to improve symptoms of depression, as it has a relaxing effect on the mind. Taking fuller breaths also provides the body with a greater supply of energy, which can be used to fuel the body's self-repair mechanisms.

The deep breathing exercise listed below can help improve your breathing and provide you with wonderful benefits. This technique involves the use of the diaphragm to breathe, which alters a person's physiology by activating the relaxation center in the brain.

1. Sit or lie comfortably in a quiet place.

2. With your feet slightly apart, place one hand on your abdomen near your navel, and the other hand on your chest.

3. Inhale through your nose and exhale through your mouth, concentrating on your breathing pattern.

4. Inhale while slowly counting to 4. As you exhale, slightly distend your abdomen, causing it to rise about one inch. You should initially feel your abdomen rise, then your chest as it fills with air.

5. As you breathe in, imagine warm or cool air flowing in and going to all parts of your body.

6. Pause for one second, then exhale slowly to a count of 4. You should notice your abdomen moving inward as you exhale.

7. As you exhale, imagine all the tension and stress leaving your body.

8. Continue this process for about 10–15 minutes.

9. Resume normal breathing if you feel faint or lightheaded.

Meditation

Meditation can be broadly defined as any activity that keeps your attention pleasantly anchored in the present moment. There are four elements common to most forms of meditation: a quiet and peaceful environment; a comfortable body position; something to focus on, like an object, a word, or breathing; and a passive, receptive attitude. Meditation typically requires 10–30 minutes, and it is most effective when practiced daily.

Regular practice of meditation can help reduce blood pressure, heart rate, respiration, anxiety and pain levels. An 18-year study published in the *American Journal of Cardiology (2005)* claims that practicing meditation can extend people's life span and reduce the risk of dying from cardiovascular disease or cancer. Researchers found that those who practiced meditation had a 23% reduction in overall death rate, a 30% reduction in cardiovascular disease death rate, and a

49% reduction in cancer death rate, when compared to those not practicing meditation.

Below is a simple technique that can be used to meditate, and thus elicit the relaxation response. The two basic components necessary to achieve this response is a mantra, a single word or syllable that is repeated over and over in a rhythmic, chant-like manner (silently or aloud), and the disregard of other thoughts that come to mind during the mantra.

1. Find a quiet, comfortable place to sit or lie down, and close your eyes.

2. Relax all your muscles.

3. Breathing through your nose, repeat silently or aloud a mantra every time you exhale.

4. When disruptive thoughts enter your mind, let them go and return to your mantra. The more you practice, the longer you'll stay focused.

5. Continue for 10–20 minutes.

6. Attempt to meditate once in the morning and again later in the day.

In addition to deep breathing exercises and meditation, you can also incorporate a little humor therapy into your daily routine. It's simple, fun and your penis will thank you. Laughter reduces cortisol (the toxic stress hormone) levels in the blood. For laughs, watch funny movies, read a humorous book, or spend time with friends or family members who make you laugh.

Other approaches to reducing stress include:

1. Keep a positive attitude. Believe in yourself. Instead of saying, "I have a problem," say, "I need a solution."

2. Accept that there are events you cannot control.

3. Be assertive instead of aggressive. "Assert" your feelings, opinions or beliefs instead of becoming angry, combative or passive. If you feel that anger is getting the best of you, write a letter to the editor of the local paper to vent your frustrations, assuming that your current peeve is a newsworthy or local-news item.

4. Exercise regularly. Your body can fight stress better when it is fit. And carrying out the garbage or clipping the hedges do not count as exercise.

Set a time aside every day specifically for structured exercise, like a hard, brisk walk at the park; weight workouts; a competitive game of basketball; or jogging around the gym's track.

5. Limit or avoid the use of alcohol and caffeine. Really. Do you need that beer? How crummy will your day be if you don't drink all that coffee for a change? Well, if it turns out to be crummy anyway, you can offset this with exercise. If you're already exercising, either do more of it, or increase intensity. If all you've been doing is walking on a treadmill, maybe it's time to start jogging.

6. Set realistic goals and expectations.

7. Get enough rest and sleep. Your body needs time to recover from stressful events. But don't overdo it. There's a such thing as a "power walk," but the term "power nap" is misleading. Too much rest is not good.

8. Don't rely on alcohol or drugs to reduce stress. Go to a boxing gym instead. Or hit some golf balls or throw some darts.

Practicing these stress-reduction techniques just a few minutes a day will do wonders for your libido and improve your sexual performance. If you find that you need a little more discipline when it comes to practicing these techniques, take a yoga or meditation class at your local fitness center.

7

Exercise for Memorable Hard-Ons

Exercise Your Body for Firmer Erections

It's a fact: Men who exercise regularly and are cardio-fit have firmer erections. Research published in the *Journal of the American Medical Association (2004)* indicates that losing weight and exercising more can improve sexual function in about one third of overweight men suffering from erectile dysfunction. In the study, researchers wanted to determine how healthy lifestyle interventions could help improve ED in obese, middle-aged men who did not have heart disease, diabetes, hypertension or other conditions known to cause ED.

Along with exercising two hours a week, half of the men studied were placed on a calorie-restrictive diet in which their average caloric intake dropped from 2,340 to about 2,000 calories daily. Their prescribed diet boosted their fiber intake, and they substituted saturated fats (like those found in commercially baked goods) with healthier monounsaturated and polyunsaturated fats (like those found in nuts or in foods specifically listing healthy fats like canola or safflower oils). The other half was not placed on any specific regimen. After two years, the men who were advised to lose weight saw little improvement—in either weight loss or sexual function. But the men who ate less and exercised more lost about 15% of their weight. More importantly, one in three regained sexual function.

Researchers concluded that sedentary men may be able to reduce their risk of ED by adopting regular physical activity at a level of at least 200 calories a day, which corresponds to walking briskly for two miles. Not a high price to pay for improved sexual function.

Exercise can also delay the onset of ED. A Harvard study involving some 31,000 men, 55 to 90 years old, found that those who regularly exercised typically had a 10-year delay in ED compared with sedentary guys. This amounts to not having to depend on medications or other ED remedies for an additional 10 years, if at all.

In addition to delaying the onset of ED, exercise will:

- help maintain or revitalize performance and satisfaction in the bedroom (or back of the car, or under that tree, or …)

- increase your sexual energy and endurance

- reduce your risk of heart disease, stroke, high blood pressure, osteoporosis (yes—as men age, they, too, are at increased risk for brittle bones—unless they take preventive measures), diabetes and obesity

- reduce your risk for cancers of the colon and prostate

- increase your life expectancy by 1–2 years. This may not seem like a whole lot, but think of it in terms of exercise adding life to your years … which means life to your penis.

"One could postulate that it would at least add years to your ability to have and maintain an erection," says researcher Eric B. Rimm, an associate professor at the Harvard School of Public Health. "Those who were physically active had a lower risk."

Rimm and his colleagues looked at data from questionnaires by 31,742 men from age 53 to 90 in the *Health Professionals Follow-up Study* of dentists, optometrists, podiatrists, pharmacists and veterinarians. The researchers excluded men with prostate cancer because impotence can be a side effect of surgery for the cancer.

The researchers checked which lifestyle and health factors affected the risk of erectile dysfunction, which the study defined as the ability to have and maintain an erection adequate for intercourse. Their findings were published in the August 2006 issue of the *Annals of Internal Medicine*.

Men who were physically active reported better erections, and the most physically active men did best. Men who were able to run at least 3 hours a week had a 30% lower risk of impotence than men who did little or no exercise. These men seemed to have the sexual ability of men two to five years younger than they were, Rimm says.

However, Rimm states there was still a 15% to 20% reduction in the risk of ED among men who were able to briskly walk 30 minutes most days of the week. This much activity is the minimum level that federal officials recommend for good health. Being a vigorous exerciser and adding other healthy lifestyle factors, such as not smoking, staying lean and drinking only moderately had the effect of adding 10 years to a man's sexual status, according to Rimm.

Exercising on a consistent basis:

- keeps joints, tendons and ligaments flexible so it's easier to move around (a bonus for readers of the *Kama Sutra*)

- reduces many of the effects of aging

- boosts the activity of the immune system

- contributes to your mental well-being and helps treat depression

- helps relieve stress and anxiety

- reduces the urge to smoke for those trying to quit

- significantly improves mental skills that decline with age

- helps maintain a normal weight by increasing your metabolism (the rate at which you burn calories)

The best form of exercise for your penis are activities that result in rhythmic physical exertion, such as swimming laps, rigorous walking, jogging, bicycling and aerobics classes (where you might even meet some attractive ladies)! Aerobic exercises create a training effect. This training effect strengthens the heart and improves lung capacity. Additionally, the hormonal system and metabolic reactions are also strengthened in their ability to cope with stressors.

One of the biggest problems we have noticed at fitness centers and gyms is that many people simply "go through the motions" during aerobic activity. It's not uncommon to see people on treadmills or bikes reading a book or watching TV and not even breaking a sweat. They've hardly increased their heart rate one beat during the entire session and are simply wasting their time. Whether you seek to improve your cardiovascular health or lose excess body fat, you must exercise hard enough to increase your heart rate. Don't be afraid to break a sweat while exercising.

To achieve the most benefits from exercise, you should engage in aerobic-type activities for at least 30–45 minutes, preferably most days of the week. Current studies suggest that at least five times a week is best. If you are a beginner, exercise for a few minutes each day and build up to 45 minutes.

Again, mowing the lawn for 45 minutes does not count. You must not let yourself get into the habit of trading planned exercise time for yard chores or household jobs like painting or sanding the baseboards. Activities of this type are nonsystematic and can actually harm your body, due to their sometimes-stressful nature, not to mention the non-neutral spinal alignment and uneven use of the body that are involved.

If you have never exercised, it may also be wise to consider hiring a certified personal trainer. A personal trainer can help you develop an exercise program that's right for you (no need to tell the trainer that your goal is enhanced penis function). The trainer can also help keep you motivated if you require a little kick in the ass to keep yourself going.

If you currently suffer from severe heart disease or some other marked medical condition, you may require a medically supervised exercise program. Speak to your doctor if you fall into this category before beginning an exercise regimen.

Exercise Your Penis

No, we're not asking that you put your penis through a workout at the gym that includes penile pushups and penile curls. When we say, "Exercise your penis," we are referring to your PC muscle (PC does not stand for "penis control muscle"). Both men and women have a PC (pubococcygeus) muscle. The next time you go to the restroom and begin urinating, try to stop your flow midway. You should feel your PC muscles contract and your anus tighten. Try stopping and starting your flow a few times until you become familiar with the function of this muscle.

Exercising your PC muscles on a regular basis can help prolong the duration of lovemaking and increase the intensity of your climax. It can also help improve the strength of your erection. Sorry guys, but exercising your penis will not help improve its length or girth.

The following penis exercises are similar to Kegel exercises that are practiced by some women to strengthen their pelvic floor muscles. In order to be effective, these exercises must be practiced frequently. The stronger your PC muscle, the more enjoyable sex will become. It won't be long before you can hang a towel over your penis and begin to raise and lower it at will. Hey, think of how impressed your wife or girlfriend will be with your new trick!

Avoid contracting your abdominal, thigh, or buttocks muscles, or squeezing your sphincter muscle only. This is something many people do, but it reduces the effectiveness of the Kegel exercise. Concentrate on breathing and trying to keep yourself relaxed, and only tense the PC muscles you are using. Try not to tense up your whole body.

The Basic Kegel

The basic Kegel can be done anytime and anywhere. Start by squeezing and holding your PC muscles for a count of 3–5 seconds, then release and relax for 5 seconds. See how many times you can do this before you feel your muscles getting tired. Most men will tire quickly, indicating the need for strengthening.

Perform Sets and Repetitions

You will get the most from your Kegel exercises if you get into performing sets of repetitions of the squeezing. The goal in performing sets and repetitions is to progressively increase the repetitions and sets of Kegels performed. If in the previous exercise, you were able to perform 10 contractions (3–5 seconds w/5-second rest periods), then 10 is your baseline. Once you have determined your baseline, perform your exercises, and every couple of days increase both the length of time you hold and squeeze, and the number of repetitions per set.

As a general guideline, work up to a point where you can hold the squeeze for 20 seconds. Then perform 3 sets of 10 repetitions. So for your first set, you would squeeze and hold for 20 seconds, relax for 20 seconds, and repeat 10 times. Continue for two more sets. As you become stronger, you can try increasing the number of repetitions, the time you squeeze and hold for, and the number of total sets performed each day. Remember not to push yourself to the point of pain or discomfort.

The Squeeze and Release

The goal of the squeeze and release is to perform as many repetitions as possible within a specific timeframe. Begin by squeezing and relaxing your PC muscle for 2 minutes a day, and gradually work your way up to doing it for 5 minutes, three times daily.

Keep in mind that because you can do these exercises just about anywhere and at any time, there is absolutely no excuse to neglect your exercises. No one will know that you're squeezing, unless of course you keep smiling like a goofball while doing them. You don't need to set aside a big chunk of time to do Kegel exercises. Do a few while waiting for a stoplight to turn green. In the last 10 minutes before lunch, when you're sitting at a desk, do a few.

Because the muscle heals quickly, you'll begin noticing that you're awakening with more solid erections, and that's always a good thing, especially if Petunia is sleeping next to you in the buff come morning (you know what I mean).

We recommend that you complete your exercises every single day for the rest of your life. Your sexual abilities and control will increase immensely, and you'll find that your penis has become stronger and firmer. Remember that the results will not be evident the instant you've done your first bunch of exercises. It takes time, like with any muscle that you begin "training" regularly.

Once you begin to master your exercises and are able to see a significant difference, the next time you're making love with your woman, stay inside her without moving. Instead of going in and out like you normally would, simply squeeze and release your PC muscle.

8

How to Feed Your Penis

Dietary Recommendations—Feed Your Penis Well

Poor dietary choices (i.e., processed foods like boxed noodle mixes or frozen dinners, fast foods, and refined foods like glazed donuts) can lead to vascular disease (the most common cause of ED), which interferes with the erection process by restricting blood flow to the penis.

Think of the blood vessels in your body as an internal plumbing system. Just as in your home, the larger pipes feed into much smaller ones, which are much more likely to clog due to their smaller diameter. The same holds true with respect to the arteries in your penis. They are some of the smaller vessels in your body and have a much higher likelihood of clogging first. When a "clog" occurs in your penile vessels (due to the accumulation of plaque on the interior vessel walls), blood flow to the penis is reduced, thus making it difficult or near impossible to maintain an erection. Researchers now know that ED may be an early warning sign of cardiovascular disease.

ED due to vascular disease may readily respond to dietary and nutritional changes aimed at promoting penile arterial health. *The Penis Diet* provides you with a proven plan to help prevent or even reverse the formation of plaques within arteries and increase blood flow to the penis. This diet can be used alone or as an adjunct to conventional treatments such as medication. Keep in mind that for this diet to be effective, you must be committed. You cannot dine on batter-dipped fish and fries, or jelly donuts and soda most days of the week, and then throw in a part-time mix of spinach salads and pears. It simply does not work that way.

Additionally, you should also not expect immediate results from this plan. ED due to vascular disease takes many years to develop. It will not improve in a few days or weeks. It may take several months before you begin to notice significant improvement in sexual function. But also realize this: Unlike medication, the results you achieve from this plan will be permanent and without side effects.

The Penis Diet will not only help improve sexual function, but just as important, it will help improve your overall health and fitness level. The proposed dietary guidelines are listed below. As you can see, they do not involve consuming a platter of exotic mammalian penises. The diet is based on some very simple guidelines.

General Dietary Guidelines

- Reduce your consumption of animal products. Yes, men, this won't be one of the easiest things you've ever done—turning down that buffalo burger—but keep reminding yourself it's all for your "manhood." Restrict protein to certain types of fish (salmon, tuna, sardines, halibut and mackerel), lean free-range meats and poultry, and eggs. Only sparingly should you consume fatty fish, red meats and dairy products.

- Increase your daily intake of whole, fresh and unprocessed foods. Plant foods, such as whole grains, fruits and vegetables, nuts and legumes, should compromise comprise the majority of your daily food volume. Include fruits (lots of richly pigmented berries to support vascular integrity), vegetables, whole grains, soy, beans, seeds, nuts, olive oil, and coldwater fish (mentioned above). Simply put, the closer to nature a food is, the better it is for you.

- Increase your intake of dietary fiber, especially the "soluble" type.

- Restrict your intake of soda, sweetened fruit drinks, candy, bakery products, cheese, milk, refined foods like white bread and bagels, fried foods, fast foods and caffeine.

- Eat less, but more often. This is called grazing. You should eat more like a gazelle, and less like a lion. A lion gorges to the point of being too full to do much more than nap for several hours, and long periods of time occur between each gorge. Gazelles or deer, on the other hand, nibble throughout the day, every day.

- Increase your intake of fresh, clean water. Drink 50% of your body weight in ounces of water daily (e.g., if you weigh 150 lbs, drink 75 oz of water daily), unless you have congestive heart failure. Have a water treatment system installed at your house. Don't assume bottled water is free of toxins. Bottled water typically comes from the same municipal water source as tap water.

Reduce Your Consumption of Animal Products

During a lifetime, the average meat eater will consume approximately 36 pigs, 36 sheep, 750 chickens and poultry, and seven cows—which translates to 4,200 pounds of beef. Animal products, including cheese, milk and eggs, play a very limited role in a healthful diet. The exception is low-fat organic yogurt with pro-biotics.

Animal products contain high amounts of saturated fat and cholesterol. When you consume animal products, you also ingest the hormones, antibiotics and other chemicals given to the animal prior to its slaughter. A diet high in animal products is also associated in one way or another with heart disease, cancer, stroke, diabetes, arthritis, constipation, obesity, gout, gallstones, kidney stones and … you guessed it, erectile dysfunction.

The Adventist Health Study found that men who consumed beef four or more times per week were twice as likely to die from heart disease as men not consuming beef. Recent findings presented at the 96th Annual Meeting of the American Association for Cancer Research (2005) revealed that people who ate more than 2 ounces of red meat or pork a day had a 50% increased risk of pancreatic cancer. The bottom line here is that a diet rich in animal products will accelerate the development of ED, and likely lead to disability and a premature death in the process.

Completely eliminating all animal products from the diet is unrealistic for most people. But you can work on cutting back on animal products, such as giving up the breakfast meats (bacon, ham, sausage) or avoiding fast-food establishments.

Now, how does one go about avoiding fast-food places? Here's a trick: Next time you're tempted to get that cheeseburger or double-decker Whopper orBig Mac, think about how it's prepared—by some teenager who bites his nails or picks at her pimples, or maybe an adult who just stuck a finger in his ear before handling the bun of your burger.

Or maybe he was picking at his moustache, or she ran her fingers through her hair, which is due for a washing. And along the way, a bit of her nail ended up in the sauce of your big jack sandwich. Who knows where fast-food hands have been right before they handled your food? People do scratch themselves, you know. Or sometimes they wipe the gunk out of their eyes. Do you think they scrub their hands with soap every time they touch their body? Bet that chili cheese dog or deluxe burger doesn't sound so appetizing anymore!

If you plan on eating dairy products, opt for no-fat or low-fat varieties. If you are hell-bent, however, on continuing to eat some bacon, ham or sausage, at least purchase it from a whole-foods mart or health food store, because these stores sell preservative-free versions of these meats. Read the ingredients list. Do not buy food that contains sodium nitrite. This is a carcinogen.

If you continue to consume red meat, always choose the leanest cuts of beef possible. Purchase organic, grass-fed beef and pork, and free-range chicken and turkey. Organic, grass-fed cattle are lower in fat, hormones, antibiotics and residue from pesticides, insecticides and herbicides commonly found in grain-fed cattle. Remember, these products may be "healthier" than their conventional counterparts, but they are still considered animal products, and as such, their consumption should be limited.

Eat More Plant Foods

The low-carb diet revolution has convinced many people that carbs are bad and that a diet rich in red meat and fat provides the path to a fit and healthy body. Unfortunately, most people following these diets are not seeing the complete picture, and endanger their health in the process. Increasing your intake of protein and fat may yield the short-term benefit of temporary weight loss (most of which is water), but ultimately, this will increase your risk for numerous conditions and diseases, including erectile dysfunction.

Maybe you know someone who lost 100 pounds from sticking to a very low-carb diet. But that weight loss is from calorie restriction, not carb restriction. After all, if your only choices for food are meat, eggs and bacon, you'll most likely end up eating a lot less than you usually do. Limited choices can get tiring. You may still be hungry, but you'll get so sick of meat that you'll end up not eating, and thereby lose weight. But this is not a good way to go about getting rid of that paunch.

By omitting or restricting the intake of certain foods or food groups, namely complex carbohydrates, from your diet, deficiencies in key nutrients and antioxidants will develop over time. People who choose a low-carb diet eliminate nature's answer to great health: plant foods. Plant foods are low in calories, fat, and sodium and contain no cholesterol. They are also rich in vitamins and minerals, essential fatty acids, antioxidants and fiber. Additionally, plant foods contain thousands of different protective phytonutrients ("phyto" means plant) that help fend off disease.

Research suggests that less than 2% of our diet should come from animal foods. In fact, studies have shown that vegetarians get far better nutrition than non-vegetarians. A plant-based diet supplies all vitamins and other nutrients like fiber adequately except for vitamin B-12, which can easily be provided in the form of a supplement. The beef and fast-food industries have convinced millions of Americans that thick hamburger patties and robust slabs of steak are necessary for a healthy diet. It's really all about money.

When it comes to the health of your penis, a diet rich in plant foods can really help "give it a lift." By eating more plant foods, you will be simultaneously reducing your consumption of animal products, including red meat, and reducing your risk for vascular disease—a major enemy of "Mr. Happy." Because plant foods tend to be much lower in calories and more filling than animal foods, achieving and maintaining an ideal body weight is accomplished with ease by adhering to a plant-based diet. The antioxidants in plant foods also help prevent the buildup of artery-clogging plaques within the vessels and maintain a healthy flow of blood to the penis.

Not only is a plant-based diet nutritionally sound, but those who follow this diet tend to be healthier and live longer than those who eat animal products on a regular basis. A 12-year study of more than 34,000 Seventh-Day Adventists in California, most of whom were vegetarians, found that on average, group members lived 10 years longer than the general population, and also remained healthier and had fewer complaints of illness than non-members.

Let's be clear: This is not the same thing as adding a few apples and some broccoli into your daily mix of lunch meats, fast-foods and other unhealthy items. It means replacing nearly all of your meals throughout the day, most days of the week, with plant foods. For example, your daily luncheon meat sandwich on white bread made with bleached flour can be replaced with peanut-butter and jam (no preservatives or additives, low-sugar/low-fat varieties) on whole-grain bread.

With that said, there are certain plant foods that are more beneficial in terms of your penis' health than others.

Oatmeal and Oat Bran

Oatmeal and oat bran are rich in soluble fiber. Soluble fiber reduces low-density lipoprotein (LDL), the "bad" cholesterol. Five to 10 grams of soluble fiber a day decreases bad cholesterol by about 5%. Lowering your LDL levels will help reduce the buildup of plaque within the arteries that supply your penis with blood, leading to firmer and longer erections.

Serving suggestion: Eating 1.5 cups of cooked oatmeal provides 4.5 grams of fiber—enough to lower your cholesterol. To mix it up a little, try oat bran, or cold cereal made with oatmeal or oat bran. You can also get oats in the form of whole-grain bread. If oatmeal is not your cup of tea, you can also try adding a fiber supplement to your daily regimen. Be sure that the supplement you choose contains a blend of soluble and insoluble fibers for best results.

Walnuts, Almonds, and More

Nuts are a rich source of healthy fatty acids (polyunsaturated). Studies have shown that walnuts can significantly reduce blood cholesterol. They also help keep blood vessels healthy and elastic. Almonds appear to have a similar effect, resulting in a marked improvement within just four weeks. A cholesterol-lowering diet in which 20% of the calories comes from walnuts may reduce bad cholesterol by 12%. For a 2,000-calorie-per-day diet, half a cup of walnuts is about 400 calories, or 20% of total calories for the day.

Serving suggestion: All nuts are high in calories, so a handful will suffice if you are trying to lose weight. As with any food, good or bad, eating too much can cause weight gain. Also, for some more variety, add chopped nuts to green salads.

Fish and Omega-3 Fatty Acids

So-called fatty fish are a rich source of omega-3 fatty acids. Studies in the 1970s showed that Greenland Eskimos had a lower rate of heart disease than other individuals living in Greenland at the same time. Analysis of dietary differences between the groups showed that the Eskimos ate less saturated fat and more omega-3 fatty acids found in fish, and whale and seal meat.

Although salmon and other fatty fish are rich sources of omega-3 fatty acids, most fish found in our markets and restaurants contain dangerously high levels of mercury and PCBs. Omega-3 fatty acids can also lower blood pressure and the risk of blood clots. In people who have already had heart attacks, fish oil—or omega-3 fatty acids—significantly reduces the risk of sudden death.

The highest levels of omega-3 fatty acids are in salmon, mackerel, lake trout, herring, sardines and albacore tuna. However, to maintain the heart-healthy benefits of fish, bake or grill it. If you can't dine with the Eskimos, other good sources of omega-3 fatty acids include flaxseed, walnuts, canola oil and soybean oil.

However, the best source for omega-3s are fish oil supplements, 1–2 grams daily. Be wary of the types of supplements used for this. Many of the commercially available products are offered in 1,000 mg capsules, BUT DO NOT HAVE 1,000 mg of DHA/EPA added together, the active omega-3 fatty acids. For this reason you may need to take up to several capsules of a particular supplement. Read the label and look at the breakdown of the fatty acids in the product. Add up the amount of DHA and EPA in the product. You should shoot for about 1,000 to 2,000 mg of DHA/EPA combined. Always read the labels for the exact amount of EPA and DHA. The ratio should be 1.6:1. An Italian study called GISSI-1 has shown that fish oil in levels of 1 gm per day can prevent a SECOND heart attack or stroke.

Berries

Berries are an excellent source of vitamins, minerals and highly potent phytochemicals, . They have also been found to possess anti-cancer and anti-heart disease properties. Increasing your intake of fresh berries, especially blueberries, can help lower cholesterol levels, regulate blood sugar levels, and reduce the risk of heart disease. Berries also promote healthy blood vessels, including the vessels in your prized organ, by limiting damage caused by free radicals.

Serving suggestion: Fresh or frozen, any berry is a great choice. You can juice berries if eating them whole is tedious. Nine ounces of blueberries, juiced, makes about 5 ounces of juice.

Legumes

Legumes include all the common beans (black, pinto, kidney, and white), lentils, fava beans, chickpeas (garbanzos), and dried split peas. There are actually 13,000 species of legumes; we, as humans, consume only 20. Legumes are rich in soluble fiber, calcium, potassium and magnesium, plus folate. Men and women who consume legumes at least four times a week have a 22% lower risk of coronary heart disease than those who consume legumes once weekly. People who consume legumes frequently (four or more times per week) have also been found to have lower blood pressure and total cholesterol, both of which are essential for healthy penile function.

Serving suggestion: Add beans to salads or eat just by themselves. Raw fava beans are surprisingly tasty. Lentil and garbanzo bean sprouts can also be enjoyed raw. If salads and raw beans are not your thing, enjoy a daily serving of bean soup.

Avocados

Avocados, nicknamed "alligator pears" because of their bumpy exteriors, got their name from the ancient Aztec word for "testicle." Maybe that is why men once believed that eating avocados would boost their virility. Avocados are loaded with healthy monounsaturated fat, potassium, fiber and antioxidants.

The avocado fights high cholesterol, high blood pressure, heart disease, diabetes, cancer and stroke. It's high in fat—30 grams per fruit, but it is mostly monounsaturated fat. This fat helps protect good HDL cholesterol, while wiping out the bad cholesterol that clogs your arteries (including those leading to the penis).

An avocado contains 10 grams of fiber, as well as a plant compound called beta-sitosterol. These both help lower cholesterol. One study from Australia demonstrated how eating half to one-and-a-half avocados a day for three weeks could lower total cholesterol by more than 8% without lowering good cholesterol. Avocados also contain more than two-and-a-half times as much potassium as a banana. Many studies show that potassium helps reduce high blood pressure.

Serving suggestion: Avocados can be enjoyed raw or as a dip (guacamole) that can be served with raw cauliflower, broccoli and carrots. They also make a great addition to fresh salads.

Dark Chocolate/Cocoa

Dark chocolate contains high amounts of cocoa, a very potent source of antioxidants. Research conducted at the University of Scranton has demonstrated that the quality and quantity of antioxidants in chocolate is relatively high when compared to other high-antioxidant foods. Cocoa powder ranks the highest of the chocolate products, followed by dark chocolate and milk chocolate.

According to the Chocolate Manufacturers Association, dark chocolate contains about eight times the polyphenol antioxidants found in strawberries. In November 2001, researchers from Pennsylvania State University found that people with a diet high in flavonoid-rich cocoa powder and dark chocolate have slightly higher concentrations of HDL when compared with the control group. In a more recent study published in the journal *Hypertension (2005),* researchers from Italy found that dark chocolate may lower blood pressure in people with high blood pressure. The research also found that levels of LDL in these individuals dropped by 10%.

Because dark chocolate exhibits favorable changes in cholesterol levels and blood pressure, it may help ward off heart and vascular disease, and in the process, protect against erectile ED. One word of caution: Although dark chocolate is healthy, this is not a license to overindulge. Chocolate is still high in calories and can add to weight gain.

Serving suggestion: If something chocolate is very dark in color, this doesn't mean it's healthy. Hostess cupcakes are very dark, but most of this is sugar and other processed fare. For health benefits, consume only minimally processed dark chocolate, which is also much lower in sugar than milk chocolate.

Extra-Virgin Olive Oil

Extra-virgin olive oil is an extremely good source of heart-healthy fat. Again, anytime you are able to improve the health of the vessels feeding blood into the penis, you reduce your odds of ED. Olive oil works its magic by lowering the bad cholesterol without affecting the good cholesterol. Olive oil contains polyphenols that further lower your risk for heart disease, as well as possibly reduce your risk for cancer, rheumatoid arthritis, diabetes, and high blood pressure.

Serving suggestion: About 2 tablespoons of olive oil is all it takes to reap the health benefits. Add to salads or as a topping on cooked vegetables.

Green Tea

Here is a giant source for disease-fighting catechins. Green tea comes from the leaves of the white-flowered tea plant, Camellia sinensis, a bush native to Asia. Catechin, a phytochemical, is the main component in green tea and is present in higher amounts than in grape juice and red wine, which are also believed to reduce the rate of heart disease. Recent research suggests that antioxidants in green tea play a role in reducing the negative effects of bad cholesterol, lowering triglyceride levels and increasing the production of good cholesterol. They have also been shown to inhibit excessive blood clotting, which helps fight heart disease and stroke.

Serving suggestion: To reap the therapeutic benefits of green tea, 4–5 cups a day must be consumed. This is made easier by steeping two teabags per cup of hot water.

Additional Tips

In general, however, simply make a valiant effort to increase your consumption of plant-based foods. Make sure these foods include those with naturally intense colors. When selecting produce, go for the purples, reds, oranges and deep, dark greens. This means all berries, plums, grapes, beets, cherries, apples, radishes, tomatoes, oranges, cantaloupes, dark green leaves and broccoli are the best ones to choose.

Eat your vegetables raw as much as possible, as in green salads more often than than stir-fried vegetables. Also, whole apples are far superior to their baked counterparts, in apple pie. Raw vegetables are superior to cooked ones, as a general rule. Some exceptions do exist, however. For example, cooked tomato products have about four times the lycopene (antioxidant) content as raw tomatoes. Cooked artichokes also rank super-high in overall antioxidant capacity. Steaming broccoli and cauliflower lightly, only to the point where they still retain their brightness, will retain some of their valuable enzymes.

But with these exceptions aside, do eat raw plant foods as much as you can, for several reasons:

1. Plants in raw form are as close to their natural state as possible.

2. Cooking destroys most of a plant's enzymes.

3. An enzyme-rich diet takes a load off of the digestive system, thus sparing energy in the body to go to work to keep disease processes in check. This, in turn, will translate to a more vigorous penis and reliable erections.

Increase Intake of Dietary Fiber

Fiber is a substance found only in plants, such as fruits, vegetables and grains. The part of the plant fiber that you eat is called dietary fiber and is an important part of a healthy diet. Dietary fiber is made up of two main types—insoluble and soluble. Both types of fiber are important in the diet and provide benefits to the digestive system by helping maintain regularity. Soluble fiber can help lower your overall blood cholesterol level and reduce levels of bad cholesterol that can cause plaque buildup in the arteries—including those supplying the penis with blood. Fiber also works to keep your body from absorbing fat and cholesterol from food. Insoluble fiber passes through your digestive tract largely intact and can help to normalize bowel movements and maintain a clean intestinal tract.

Aim for a daily fiber intake of 25–30 grams, one-quarter of which should be the soluble type. The average American currently consumes only 3–4 grams of soluble fiber daily. Increasing your intake of fruits and vegetables, nuts and seeds, legumes, oats and barley can help ensure an optimal level of fiber. Soluble fiber is found in oats, peas, beans, certain fruits, and psyllium. If you find it hard to consume enough fiber from diet alone, then a fiber supplement is a good option. Be sure that it contains a mixture of both soluble and insoluble fiber and is free of added sugars.

Reduce Consumption of the "White Death"

The average American consumes over 150 pounds of added sugars each year, according to the Center for Science in Public Interest. Sweetened soft drinks, sweetened fruit juices, breakfast cereals and snack foods are major contributors to dietary sugar. Even some soups contain sugar, and that is mm, mm, bad! (If you've ever wondered how that popular brand of tomato soup, for instance, could taste so amazingly good and sweet … read the ingredients, and you'll find out!)

The term "sugar" includes: corn syrup, molasses, maltodexterin and any word ending in "-ose," such as lactose and fructose. *The Penis Diet* widens the term "sugar" to include all refined carbohydrates, such as white rice, white bread, enriched flours, sugary cereals and pasta made from white flour.

Every time you consume sugar, insulin levels in your blood increase. Insulin removes sugar from the blood and transports it to the cells, where it is stored as fat. Chronically elevated insulin levels can lead to cardiovascular disease, diabetes and ultimately, erectile dysfunction, due to hardened and plaque-filled arteries leading their way to the penis. There's nothing sweet about that.

Guidelines for Reducing Sugar Intake

- Don't be fooled by those commercials showing "moms" serving their kids some brightly colored drink that's high in vitamin C. Manufacturers market these beverages as great sources of vitamin C when, in reality, they are nothing more than fruit-flavored sugar water.

- Beware of specialty coffee drinks. They can be a significant source of sugar.

- Replace sugary breakfast cereals with whole grain cereals that are lower in sugar (again, read the labels).

Consume Smaller Meals More Often

When it comes to dropping weight or maintaining a healthy body weight, eating four to six smaller meals and snacks each day is the only way to go. Research has found that people who eat smaller, more frequent meals have consistently lower cholesterol levels than people who consume larger meals less often. Lower cholesterol levels amount to healthier blood vessels, including those leading to and supplying the penis.

Although it seems counter-intuitive, eating more often—not less often—actually helps control weight. Studies have demonstrated that those who eat four to six smaller meals per day have less body fat than those consuming two or three meals daily, despite the fact that both groups take in about the same amount of calories.

Eating increases your metabolic rate (the rate at which you burn calories) because it takes energy to break down and digest food. As mentioned previously, consuming only one or two meals a day actually fools your body into thinking that it's in a state of starvation, and thus, metabolism slows. You can crank it up by eating several smaller meals more frequently. Because your body's metabolic rate has a natural cycle of highs and lows, peaking late in the day and dropping to its lowest point during sleep, you should avoid large meals late at night, especially right before bedtime.

Eating one or two larger big meals rather than five or six smaller meals and snacks throughout the day can also impact energy levels. Consuming a big, robust meal can cause your blood sugar level to rise quickly and then fall, leading to fatigue and sleepiness. This is one reason you should not consume a big meal before engaging in sexual activity. Think about how many times you have been overcome with extreme sleepiness shortly after eating one of those big, man-portioned TV dinners. Spacing out smaller meals and snacks throughout the day helps your body avoid dramatic fluctuations in blood sugar, and it also improves energy level and performance.

For some, switching to smaller, more frequent meals is relatively easy. For others, it can be a hassle, as well as an exercise in humility. What man wants to be seen eating like a woman? (Though some women eat like bears.) Keep in mind that you don't have to actually consume four, five or six entire meals every few hours; you just have to eat something healthful such as a serving of fruit or a handful of nuts. The best way to accomplish this is to eat three normal, but smaller meals, with snacks in between. Once you regularly eat this way, you will begin to notice the benefits, including a satisfied feeling throughout the day and greater success with portion control. Your energy level will be consistent, and you will avoid those late afternoon slumps.

Drink More Clean Water

Your body consists of approximately 70% water. So vital is water to survival that you could not function more than a few days without it. By contrast, you could survive up to six weeks without food. Supplying your body with plenty of fresh, clean water each day is essential for optimal health and functioning.

Seventy-five percent of Americans are chronically dehydrated. This doesn't mean they always feel thirsty. In fact, you can be dehydrated, yet not be thirsty. To prevent dehydration, you'll need to drink water when you're not thirsty at all. Dehydration can lead to an increase in the stress hormone cortisol. Increases in cortisol can lead to weight gain over time, as it impairs the body's ability to burn fat. Studies have also found that elevated cortisol levels can decrease testosterone levels in the body and lead to a reduced sex drive and erectile dysfunction.

Drinking more water can also help reduce appetite. In 37% of all Americans, their thirst mechanism is so weak, it is mistaken for hunger. A study from the University of Washington in 2002 found that one glass of water shut down midnight hunger pangs for almost 100% of dieters examined.

Many authorities recommend drinking approximately 1/2 ounce of water per pound of body weight. This means that a 140 lb. individual would require about 70 ounces, or about nine cups of water, per day. If you are active, the recommendation is even higher. A simple means for assessing your hydration status is by checking the color of your urine. Very light to clear-colored urine indicates that you are likely well-hydrated. Dark urine can be an indication of dehydration and a signal to drink more water.

We recommend sipping on spring, purified or filtered water throughout the day. Also keep in mind that many beverages such as coffee, tea and juice contain water that counts toward your daily consumption. Conditions like diabetes and congestive heart failure will not fare well with so much fluid, so coordinate this with your physician first to avoid a trip to the ER.

So how does water intake relate to penile health? Keep in mind that erectile dysfunction can be caused by being overweight*, high blood pressure, diabetes and stress. Dehydration can lead to an increase in the stress hormone cortisol. This, in turn, can lead to weight gain over time, as it impairs the body's ability to burn fat. Weight gain points to a higher chance of getting diabetes or high blood pressure, and we already know that these two conditions are often precursors to an uncooperative penis.

Elevated cortisol levels can also decrease testosterone levels in the body, and a man walking around with reduced testosterone is a man walking around wondering why he can't get it up when Misty is around. Chronic dehydration can lead to weight gain, which in turn can lead to hypertension and diabetes. Chronic dehydration can lead to increased production of stress hormones, which can also lead to ED.

Bottom line: Drink your water! Every day! Thirsty or not! And soda does not count toward your water quota of eight glasses a day.

Simple Suggestions

Begin your new eating plan today by first going through your refrigerator and cabinets and ridding yourself of all unhealthy food items. These may include processed and convenience foods, luncheon meats, cured meats, all foods containing hydrogenated oils, baked goods, and foods high in sugar. Your body will indeed thank you for it!

And once again, here is a simple rule to follow: "The closer to nature a food is, the better it is for you."

Next, head to the market or your local health food store and stock up on the antioxidant-rich fruits and vegetables, whole grains and healthy beverages mentioned throughout this chapter. As you consume healthy foods and beverages, visualize your body sailing closer toward optimal health and farther away from illness and disease. At all times, you should view your body as a finely tuned engine. Feed it well and it will run well for a very long time. Feed it poorly, and you'll be spending plenty of time for repairs at doctors' offices and hospitals.

9

Nutritional Supplementation for Your Penis

There are a number of nutritional supplements that can actually increase blood flow to the penis or increase the nitric oxide needed to sustain erections. Although these supplements do not cure ED, they can provide a natural alternative or adjunct to pharmaceutical options. It is important to remember that these supplements do not *cause* erections; they just make it easier to sustain one when sexually aroused.

The FDA reviews all prescription drugs for safety. Supplements are under no such review. None have been reviewed for effectiveness. None for safety. None for quality or quantity. This presents a quandary. Surely these natural substances that have been used for possibly hundreds or thousands of years can't hurt us. Right?

Well, true believer, you are wrong. Even too much water can harm us. Remember this mantra: *Everything in moderation!*

Supplements are intended to provide nutritional support. Because a supplement or a recommended dose may not be appropriate for all persons, a physician (i.e., a licensed naturopathic physician or holistic MD or DO) should be consulted before using any product to treat ED.

Daily Multivitamin Supplement with Minerals

A daily multivitamin will help offset the health risks associated with an inadequate diet—and even many people who think they eat a "healthy" diet can be missing out on an lot of important nutrients. One study estimated the potential preventative health benefits of multivitamin supplementation in the elderly at $1.6 billion over the following five years.

The authors of the study calculated these savings on improved immune functioning and a reduction in the relative risk of coronary artery disease. Taking a daily multivitamin may also help protect against damage caused by free radicals. Remember, both coronary artery disease and free radical damage can contribute to erectile dysfunction. No scientific data has demonstrated harm in taking a daily multivitamin, so safety should not be a concern.

When choosing a multivitamin formula, be sure it contains a minimum of 100% of the daily values for each nutrient. Additionally, choose a multivitamin with minerals, since most Americans tend to be deficient as a result of depleted mineral stores in the soil and the extensive refinement of food. To maximize absorption, take your daily multivitamin/mineral supplement with a meal, preferably breakfast.

Niacin (Nicotinic Acid): This is vitamin B3.

Penis benefits: Improves blood flow to your penis due to the vitamin's positive effect on the cardiovascular system, and keeps penile blood vessels free of artery-clogging plaques which can hinder the flow of blood to the penis, and lead to ED. Think of niacin as an oral form of "Liquid Plumber" that travels through and cleans out the "internal pipes" of your body to keep them healthy. At present, there are no drugs that can offer the cardiovascular benefits of niacin.

After analyzing data from more than 83,000 heart patients who participated in 23 different clinical trials, researchers at the University of Washington found that a regimen that increased HDL by 30% and lowered LDL by 40% in the average patient would reduce the risk of heart attack or stroke by 70%. In 1975, a landmark study of more than 8,000 men who had suffered heart attacks revealed that niacin was the only treatment among five tested that prevented second heart attacks. Those on niacin had a 26% reduction in heart attacks and a 27% reduction in strokes.

Dose: 1–2 grams daily. The main side effect of niacin is flushing of the skin. This effect becomes less pronounced with time, and often it can be avoided by taking the vitamin before bed with a bit of low-fat food. It can also help to start with small doses and work up to larger ones. As always, you should speak to your doctor before taking niacin, especially if you currently suffer from diabetes or heart disease.

Antioxidants

As mentioned earlier, these are free-radical busters, particularly vitamins E and C, plus the mineral selenium. Penis benefits: These improve blood circulation and blood vessel health in the penis, due to their positive effects on the cardiovascular system.

Dose: Vitamin E (alpha-tocopherol): 400 IU/day; Vitamin C: 500 mg/day; Selenium: 200 mcg/day

There are many other antioxidants available in supplement form. These include vitamin A, co-enzyme Q10, glutathione, alpha lipoic acid, grape seed extract and pycnogenol. Rather than spending your hard-earned dollars on each of these antioxidants, it's best to obtain additional antioxidant protection from dietary sources.

The foods with the highest concentration of antioxidants, in order of highest to lowest, are small red beans, wild blueberries, kidney beans, pinto beans, cultivated blueberries, cranberries, cooked artichoke hearts, blackberries, prunes, raspberries, red delicious apples, Granny Smith apples, pecans, russet potatoes (with skins), and black beans.

L-Arginine

Of all the nutritional supplements aimed at improving ED, L-arginine (an amino acid) is one of the better choices.

Penis benefits: Dilation of blood vessels necessary for a normal erection depends on nitric oxide, and nitric oxide formation depends on arginine. Studies show that arginine supplementation is particularly effective at improving ED in men with abnormal nitric oxide metabolism. L-arginine has also been found to have a direct scavenging effect on harmful free radicals and can help prevent blood clots and improve the stability of the lining of blood vessels, including those leading to and supplying the penis.

Dose: 1–2 grams per day in divided doses. For best results, try taking a dose 30 minutes before sexual activity.

Zinc Picolinate:

Zinc is a mineral that is vital to optimal function of the body.

Penis benefits: Zinc supplementation has been shown to reduce the size of the prostate and BPH (benign prostate enlargement) symptoms. Zinc may also help reduce the risk or progression of prostate cancer. There is clinical evidence indicating that cancerous prostate cells contain less zinc than healthy prostate cells. Significant depletion of zinc, associated with long-term use of diuretics, plus diabetes, digestive disorders, and certain kidney and liver diseases, has been shown to lead to erectile dysfunction in some men due to its effects on the prostate gland. Men with a history of BPH have been found to have almost a 20% increased risk of ED.

Dose: 50 mg daily

DHEA

DHEA is a hormone, the most abundant steroid in the body, and is involved in the manufacture of testosterone and other hormones.

Penis benefits: In one double-blind trial, 40 men with low DHEA levels and ED were given 50 mg DHEA per day for six months. Significant improvement in both ED and interest in sex occurred in the men taking DHEA, but not in those taking a placebo. Low blood levels of the hormone DHEA have been reported in some men with ED. Maximal concentrations of endogenous DHEA are reached in the third decade of life; then, there is a slow, steady decline of 2% per year, reaching a level of 10–20% during the eighth decade.

Dose: 50 mg per day.

Herbal Support

Herbal medicines usually do not have significant side effects when used appropriately and at suggested doses. Occasionally, an herb at the prescribed dose causes stomach upset or a headache. This may reflect the impurity of the preparation or added ingredients, such as synthetic binders or fillers. For this reason, it is recommended that only high-quality products be used. As with all medications, more is not better, and overdosing can lead to serious illness and even death.

Panax Ginseng

Asian ginseng (Panax ginseng) has traditionally been used as a supportive herb for male potency.

Penis benefits: A double-blind trial showed that 1,800 mg per day of Asian ginseng extract for three months helped improve libido and the ability to maintain an erection in men with ED. The benefit of Asian ginseng was also confirmed in another double-blind study, in which 900 mg of a concentrated extract three times a day was given for eight weeks. At the study's conclusion, researchers noted that the men in the Korean red ginseng group scored significantly better on the Mean International Index of Erectile Function than patients who received a placebo. In addition, the ginseng group scored higher on questions dealing with maintaining an erection, and 60% of the patients reported that ginseng improved erection.

Researchers noted that penile tip rigidity was also significantly improved among participants during ginseng treatment compared to placebo. Ginseng is of benefit to men with ED because it helps boost the conversion of L-arginine to nitric oxide. The most common side effects are nervousness and excitation (not something you need when you are preparing for sex).

Dose: 900–1,500 mg of concentrated extract daily.

Ginkgo Biloba

Ginkgo is probably the oldest living tree species, dating back to more than 200 million years. The use of gingko has been documented for over 1,000 years.

Penis benefits: Ginkgo biloba may help men with ED by increasing blood flow to the penis. Ginkgo's circulation enhancer, called *terpene lactone*, also significantly enhances the production of dopamine, adrenaline and other neurotransmitters in the brain, which are responsible for improved pleasure, arousal and alertness. One double-blind trial found improvement in men taking 240 mg per day of a standardized Ginkgo biloba extract (GBE) for nine months. A preliminary trial, involving 30 men who were experiencing ED as a result of medication use (selective serotonin reuptake inhibitors and other medications), found that approximately 200 mg per day of Ginkgo biloba extract had a positive effect on sexual function in 76% of the men.

Possible drug interactions: alprazolam, aspirin, diacritic, haloperidol, ibuprofen, nifedipine, omeprazole, trazodone, and warfarin. These interactions could be deadly, so be sure to discuss ginkgo with your physician if you are on any of these drugs. Adverse reactions consist of headache, dizziness, heartbeat irregularities, skin reactions and stomach upset.

Dose: 100 mg of a standardized Ginkgo biloba extract (24% ginkgo flavonglycosides) three times a day.

Yohimbine

Yohimbine is a substance found in the bark of the yohimbe tree.

Penis benefits: Yohimbe stimulates blood flow to the penis. Yohimbe has also been shown to increase libido and decrease the period between ejaculations. Yohimbe may also have a positive effect on impotence problems caused by depression. Yohimbine has been shown in several double-blind trials to help treat men with ED. Yohimbe dilates blood vessels and may help, regardless of the cause of ED.

Dose: A tincture of yohimbe bark is often used in the amount of 5 to 10 drops three times per day. Standardized yohimbe extracts are also available. A typical daily amount of yohimbine is 15 to 30 mg. It is best to use yohimbe and yohimbine under the supervision of a physician. There is a relatively small dosing range. Below a certain range, the herb doesn't work, and above it, the herb is toxic. Side effects of normal dosages include dizziness, anxiety, hyperstimulation, and nausea. As little as 40 mg a day can cause a severe drop in blood pressure, abdominal pain, fatigue, hallucinations, and paralysis.

Saw Palmetto

Saw palmetto is an herbal product commonly used in the treatment of symptoms related to benign prostatic hyperplasia (enlarged prostate). The active component is found in the fruit of the American dwarf palm tree. Studies have demonstrated the effectiveness of saw palmetto in reducing symptoms associated with benign prostatic hyperplasia.

Penis benefits: Saw palmetto stimulates a low libido and increases sexual energy. It reduces the conversion of testosterone into dihydrotestosterone (DHT). Increased levels of testosterone can help increase sex drive and improve mood.

Dose: 160 mg of the saw palmetto extract standardized to contain 85–95% fatty acids and sterols, twice daily.

Cordyceps

This is a black, blade-shaped fungus found on the Tibetan plateau of China. It has been used for its benefits in improving energy, lifespan and quality of life.

Penis benefits: It can affect many organ systems of the body and has been used in Chinese medicine for sexual dysfunction. There are a number of animal and human clinical studies to document the benefits of using certain strains of this wild plant. Results for improvement were clinically significant and better than placebo in restoring sex drive and function. It may work via the hormonal system or directly on the brain or sex organs.

Dose: There are no accurate dosing charts or instructions available. The potential side effects could be mild nausea, upset stomach and dry mouth. It is not considered to be a cancer-causing agent.

Damiana

A Mexican shrub also found in the southern U.S. and South America, this plant has quite a bit of scientific data, going back 100 years or more. Use of the plant actually began in the Mayan culture for dizziness.

Penis benefits: In the last 100 years, it has been used as an aphrodisiac, which affects desire, but not performance. The "flower power" generation brought the compound into the current age for just such an action. Unfortunately, there has been no scientific data generated to support any of these claims. There are no studies documenting effectiveness.

Dose: There is no information on appropriate dosage or side effects.

Deer Velvet

This is harvested from the surface of deer antlers, specifically the Cervus species (North American elk and red deer). It can be distributed as a powder, extract, tea, capsule or tablet after being frozen and dried, and then "manufactured."

Penis benefits: In Chinese medicine, the use of the velvet dates back over 2,000 years as an elixir to restore health and vitality (it sure worked for the deer), and to reduce swelling and treat impotence. In 1999, the use of this substance was scientifically substantiated by research according to FDA guidelines for arthritis. Interestingly enough, there is some evidence it can benefit those with immune system illnesses and circulation problems (right up the alley of ED).

Dose: 2–6 capsules of 215 mg each daily.

Possible drug interactions: There has been a report of an interaction with morphine with a development of tolerance to the drug's pain-killing properties. There have been no reported toxicity concerns.

Horny Goat Weed

Wow, what a name for a product! This has been used in traditional Chinese medicine for improving sexual performance (couldn't see that coming, could you?) and energy. Unfortunately there are no clinical trials to confirm these properties. There is no data on toxicity, either.

Rhodiola

This flowering plant grows in the sandy soil of the arctic areas of Europe and Asia. It has been used for many different ailments, including fertility problems.

Penis benefits: It has been shown in studies to stimulate neurotransmitters in the brain like norepinephrine, dopamine, serotonin (sound familiar?) and can improve the ability of these chemicals to pass into the brain. It sounds very much like an antidepressant, so it is likely better for the libido as opposed to ED.

Dose: While some studies recommend 200–600 mg/day, there is no data to support its use for ED.

Choosing the Right Regimen

Below you will find two regimens, with each containing a variety of vitamins, minerals, herbs and dietary factors. The Level I program has been designed to be used as a preventative program for those concerned about the future health of their penis. We know that many people enjoy "living for the day." However, this may be the one exception to that rule!

Our Level II regimen is more aggressive in terms of the number of products and the recommended doses for each. This program is for those who currently suffer from ED and who are looking for a nutritional supplementation program that will give them the best chance for success. Our Level II program can be used independently or as an adjunct to traditional medical care, including many of the oral medications.

Keep in mind that these regimens will not work overnight! ED is a condition that develops over years or decades. It may take several weeks or months before you begin to notice an improvement in your condition.

Our nutritional supplementation program has been designed to target both the cause and the symptoms of ED. Drugs only target the symptoms of the condition and do nothing to actually improve the health of your penis. The recommended doses below are daily amounts. Taking higher or more frequent doses will not offer better or faster results, so save your money. The recommended doses are based on scientific trials involving hundreds of thousands of subjects. You do not need to conduct your own study using higher doses.

When it comes to adding DHEA, L-Arginine, Ginseng, Ginkgo biloba and Yohimbe to your daily regimen, you should start slowly with only one product added at a time to check for side effects and results. Using L-Arginine for instance, for 1–2 weeks, and noticing an improvement may make you stop before adding other agents.

Level I—Preventative Nutritional Supplementation (Daily)

1. Daily multivitamin supplement with minerals: Dose: As directed on label.

2. Antioxidants: vitamin C (500 mg), vitamin E (400 IU), selenium (200 mcg)

3. Zinc picolinate: (50 mg)

4. Niacin: (500–1,000 mg—avoid sustained or time-release forms)

5. Omega-3 fatty acids: (1,000–2,000 mg of DHA/EPA)

6. Fiber supplement: (20–25 grams)

Level II—Therapeutic Nutritional Supplementation (Daily)

1. Daily multivitamin supplement with minerals: Dose: As directed on label.

2. Antioxidants: vitamin C (500 mg), vitamin E (400 IU), selenium (200 mcg)

3. Zinc picolinate: (50 mg)

4. Niacin: (1,000–2,000 mg—avoid sustained or time-release forms)

5. Omega-3 fatty acids: (1,000–2,000 mg of DHA/EPA)

6. DHEA: (50 mg)

7. L-Arginine: (1,000–2,000 mg twice daily)

8. Panax ginseng: (1,000–2,000 mg of concentrated extract)

9. Ginkgo biloba: (100 mg of standardized extract three times daily)

10. Yohimbe: (15–30 mg of standardized extract under physician supervision)

11. Fiber supplement: (25–30 grams/7–10 grams of soluble fiber)

Common-Sense Measures

Because most alternative and complementary treatments are not regulated, it is difficult to know just what you are getting. Here are some tips to follow when considering using herbal remedies.

• Talk to your doctor about any nutritional products you are considering before trying them, especially if you suffer from a medical condition.

• If you experience side effects such as nausea, vomiting, rapid heartbeat, anxiety, insomnia, diarrhea, or skin rashes, stop taking the herbal product and notify your doctor.

• Avoid preparations made with more than one herb.

• Beware of commercial claims of what herbal products can do. Look for scientific-based sources of information.

• Select brands carefully. Only purchase brands that list the herb's common and scientific name, the name and address of the manufacturer, a batch and lot number, expiration date, dosage guidelines, and potential side effects.

10

Additional Treatment Options

Have More SEX!

One of the best ways to improve sexual function (and your overall health) is to have more sex! The old adage, "Use is or lose it," has some truth to it.

Benefits of Having Regular Sex

- Increased life expectancy: A study published in the *British Medical Journal (1997)* found that men who reported the highest frequency of orgasm enjoyed a death rate half that of the laggards.

- Reduced risk of heart disease: In a follow-up to the study mentioned above, researchers found that having sex three or more times weekly reduced the risk of heart attack and stroke in men by 50%.

- Weight loss and improved overall fitness: Having sex three times weekly is the equivalent of running 75 miles over the course of one year. A vigorous bout of sex typically burns about 200 calories, which is about the same as running 15 minutes on a treadmill. Like exercise, sex also increases the pulse rate from about 72 bpm to 150 bpm and can improve cardiorespiratory fitness. Muscular contractions during sex can improve strength and muscle tone. Sex also increases the production of testosterone, which can help build strong bones and muscles, and helps transport DHEA, a hormone important to the functioning of the body's immune system.

- Stress relief: Sex can help relieve stress and tension and help you relax. During orgasm, the hormone oxytocin is released. Oxytocin helps will reduce stress, regulate blood pressure and temperature, relieve pain, and promote the healing of wounds.

- Pain relief: During orgasm, levels of the hormone oxytocin surge to five times the normal level. This in turn releases endorphins, which are often referred to as the body's "feel good" hormones. Endorphins can help alleviate many types of pain.

- Improved prostate health: A study published in the *Journal of the American Medical Association* found that men in their 20s who ejaculated more than five times a week were one-third less likely to develop aggressive prostate cancer than men who ejaculated four to seven times a month.

- Less-frequent cold and flu: Having sex one to two times weekly has been shown to increase the levels of an antibody called immunoglobulin A by 30 %. Increasing immunoglobulin A levels helps improve the activity of the immune system and also fends off colds and viruses.

As you can see, regular sex has many healthy benefits. By lowering your risk for cardiovascular disease, reducing stress, and improving your overall fitness level, you are inadvertently reducing your risk for erectile dysfunction and a less-than-stellar performance in the sack. To achieve the greatest benefit from sexual activity, aim for a minimum of one to two sessions weekly. If you are currently without a partner (or an unwilling partner), try masturbation, which can help produce many of the same benefits as regular sex.

Hypnosis

ED that cannot be linked to physical causes has been successfully treated by hypnosis. In one trial, three hypnosis sessions per week that were later decreased to one per month, over a six-month period, led to improvement in 75% of men in the trial. Hypnosis does require one to surrender control in order for the session to be successful.

Some men may be too full of pride to actually allow this to occur. Pride goeth before the fall (of the penis here), so humility goes a long way. In a hypnosis session, I use positive suggestion and imagery to encourage the client to overcome fears or anxieties and imagine how he can eliminate his problems. It might consist of a more positive body or self-image. It might promote confidence in approaching difficulties at work or with the opposite (or same) sex. Imagining increased blood flow and a positive body image can go a long way toward improving ED.

Acupuncture

Acupuncture might be of some benefit for men with ED. Electroacupuncture, which is acupuncture accompanied by electrical stimulation, was performed on various acupuncture in men with ED in a preliminary trial of men subjects with this condition. Two treatments were administered every week for one month. An improvement in the quality of erection was observed in 15% of the participants, and an increase in sexual activity was reported by 31% of the men. Controlled trials with larger groups of men are necessary to better test the efficacy of acupuncture therapy for men suffering from ED.

Aromatherapy

Dr. Alan Hirsch and his colleague Dr. Jason Gruss, of the Smell and Taste Research Foundation, conducted a study to investigate the impact of various aromas upon sexual response in the human male. The results of the study indicated that the combined odor of lavender and pumpkin pie had the greatest effect, increasing median penile blood flow by 40%. Next in effectiveness was the combination of black licorice and doughnut aromas, which increased arousal by 31.5%, and so on, all the way down to cranberry, which only increased penile blood flow by 2%.

So what does all this mean? This research indicates that there is a direct connection between odors and sexual response, and that it may be possible to improve sexual function using various aromas or combinations of aromas. We suggest lighting a lavender or pumpkin pie candle before sexual activity. It may be even more beneficial to burn both simultaneously, as the research indicates.

11

Final Thoughts

You may be wondering why, throughout this entire discussion so far, we have not quoted any real-life sufferers of erectile dysfunction. After all, don't books about medical conditions usually contain a number of case histories, including quoted statements from actual patients? Of course.

But if you have ED, you already know how humiliating it can make you feel, and this condition is not something that many men are willing to step forward to talk about. There are many myths and stigmas attached, and it's probably the most least openly discussed medical condition out there.

We were lucky, however, in that someone was willing to share with us his experiences with ED. And as you'll see, this patient was not atypical, in that he delayed seeking treatment. If you have ED, you will surely relate to his story, and if you are not able to identify with the end of his story, that's because you have not yet embarked on following the guidelines in this book.

We hope that by following our guidelines, this book you will help you regain what you may have lost, keep what you have, and help you to be more successful in your search for "Happy"-ness. If you do not have ED at all and have read this book just out of curiosity or to determine how you can maintain your current penis health, then do read the case history below anyway, so you can see what a healthy way of living can protect you from.

My Personal Story

I'm a 53-year-old man who suffered from erectile dysfunction for more than two years before finally being able to gather the courage to seek professional help for my condition. Prior to getting help, ED affected nearly every facet of my life, including my abil-

ity to maintain a normal relationship, my productivity at work, and my social interactions with friends and co-workers.

I avoided seeking professional help sooner out of embarrassment and shame. Rather than face the problem, I choose to just ignore my partner's sexual advances and avoid situations which had the potential to lead to sexual activity. This soon began to lead to issues with trust, intimacy and closeness, as you might expect. The fear of sexual failure caused me to withdraw emotionally and physically from my partner. It wasn't long before I was being accused of infidelity, which was the furthest thing from the truth. My productivity at the office also diminished due to a lack of self-esteem and confidence. I also began to isolate myself from my co-workers and friends.

It wasn't long before my girlfriend of three years decided enough was enough and threatened to end our relationship. It was only at this point that I decided to face the problem and seek professional help. One of the things that surprised me most was how well my doctor understood and handled things. He actually made me feel very at ease speaking about my conditions, and explained that ED affects a whole lot of men, even those in their early 20s, and that I had nothing to be embarrassed about.

In additional to prescribing me medication and specific lifestyle changes, he also stressed the importance of open communication with my partner, and told me that the first step towards successful treatment is a willingness on the part of both partners to acknowledge and discuss the problem.

I should also mention that in addition to almost ruining my life, ED may have also saved it. After ordering an array of diagnostic tests, my doctor informed me that I had advanced cardiovascular disease. ED can be an early warning sign of vascular disease. My doctor informed me that while it may seem as though my condition developed over the course of a few years, it actually began many years before my symptoms actually arose, which is not surprising, considering my unhealthy lifestyle.

My diet consisted primarily of high-fat, high-sugar processed and convenience foods. I led a sedentary lifestyle and was overweight, and was a smoker for many years. My blood pressure was also elevated, as were my cholesterol levels. My doctor informed me that each of these habits and conditions contribute to ED in one way or another by damaging penile blood vessels and restricting the flow of blood into the penis.

It was a combination of losing one of the people who meant the most to me in my life, and actually succumbing to an early death due to a heart attack or stroke, that made me actually want to change the way I live. I began to educate myself on healthy lifestyle habits and implement these changes into my daily routine. My doctor also provided me with a copy of "The Penis Diet" as a reference for natural treatment options in addition to the medication I have been prescribed. He told me that the medication would only address the symptoms of ED, but not the actual causes. The approach outlined in the book was meant to address the causes of ED.

It has only been about three months, but I feel as if I have reclaimed my life. My relationship is better than ever, and my self-esteem and confidence have improved considerably. My overall mood is upbeat and happy. If you currently suffer from ED, I can't encourage you enough to speak to your partner about it and seek professional help. Help is readily available. You just have to want it. T. B. Philadelphia, PA

As we end this discussion, remember that we have focused on improving erectile dysfunction by maintaining health and reversing diseases that are linked to the condition. Research has proven that one of the best ways to combat ED is by treating your body correctly, with respect and care. It truly is your temple. Exercise and proper diet are the cornerstones to a happy, healthy life (and penis).

We all want to live a long time, but of what use is it be 90 years old with the blindness of diabetes and blocked arteries from cigarettes? The time to begin being health-conscious is in childhood, but as we know, if you are reading this book, you are not a child. The sooner you are able to change unhealthy eating and living habits, the better off you will be. If diabetes or heart disease—or some other condition—already afflicts you, you still have a chance to make a difference and regain what has been lost.

APPENDIX A

The Penis Power Eating Plan

Ancient man probably never experienced erectile dysfunction. Penis problems were probably non-existent before the invention of processed and fried foods, transfats, white sugar, and sodium-soaked canned vegetables. In fact, according to fossil records, the diseases that plague modern man were rare during primitive times. What is the main difference between early hunter-gathererers and modern-day suit-and-tie men? Eating habits.

Yes, sir, eating habits. Today's man does not eat the way the human body has evolved. We basically evolved on untainted, all-natural meat, free of antibiotics, hormones and pesticides (livestock ingest pesticides when it eats grains; and those chemicals end up in your body). However, early man couldn't always take down a 500-pound beast with primitive weapons. Thus, he ate whatever he could get his foraging hands on: fruits, vegetation, nuts and seeds—all pure, no pesticides. And that was his diet: plant life, with some meat here and there.

Look what we've done to ourselves! Today's man is on the go and grabs whatever he can get his foraging hands on: the greasy bag handed to him from the drive-through window of the local fast-food joint; candy from the vending machine; the sugar-loaded latte from the coffee shop, accompanied by a sugar-and trans-fat-loaded pastry. No wonder erectile dysfunction cripples so many men, including those under 50. Coincidence?

If you have ED or are concerned about developing it, look no further than what you put into your mouth every day. It's really simple to grasp: A poor diet can lead to vascular disease, which is the No. 1 cause of impotence. "Vascular" pertains to blood vessels. Diseased blood vessels can't deliver adequate blood to your penis. Insufficient blood supply equals a deflated balloon of a penis. The Standard American Diet (SAD) causes plaque buildup on arterial walls. Arteries transport blood to the penis. Arterial walls caked with disgusting plaque will restrict precious blood flow to this vital organ! A prescription drug isn't always the answer to this, especially if you don't have medical coverage for these expensive pills.

So what to do? Change the way you eat before you do anything else! And don't fret; this isn't rocket science; we have it laid out crystal-clear for you right here—a sample seven-day menu plan to get your started on your way to firm, vigorous erections, enjoying the very performance you thought you'd never have again. And if you currently don't have ED, then adhering to *The Penis Diet*, along with our other recommendations, such as exercise adherence, nutritional supplementation and no smoking, will ensure that your manhood will always come through for you, anytime you desire, no matter where you are.

The Penis Power Eating Plan

MONDAY	
BREAKFAST	4 EGG WHITES 1 SLICE WHOLE GRAIN TOAST 1 APPLE 8 OZ POMEGRANATE JUICE GREEN TEA OR BLACK COFFEE
LUNCH	LARGE GARDEN SALAD W/ BABY SPINACH, TOMATO, BROCCOLI, AVOCADO, ALMOND SLIVERS EXTRA-VIRGIN OLIVE OIL AND VINEGAR DRESSING 2 SLICED HARD-BOILED EGGS OR EGG WHITES
DINNER	8 OZ BAKED OR GRILLED WILD SALMON W/ LEMON & HERBS FRESH SPINACH W/ GARLIC AND EXTRA-VIRGIN OLIVE OIL SMALL GARDEN SALAD 1 GLASS RED WINE GREEN TEA OR BLACK COFFEE 4 OZ DARK CHOCOLATE

TUESDAY	
BREAKFAST	WHEY PROTEIN SHAKE W/ 2 TABLESPOONS FIBER AND FLAX SEED 1 CUP SOY MILK 1 CUP FRESH STRAWBERRIES 8 OZ LOW-SODIUM V8 JUICE GREEN TEA OR BLACK COFFEE
LUNCH	6 OZ TUNA OR CHICKEN SALAD 2 SLICES WHOLE GRAIN BREAD 1 APPLE
DINNER	6 OZ GRILLED ORGANIC FILLET W/ ALL VISIBLE FAT TRIMMED SWEET POTATO W/ LIGHT BUTTER BROCCOLI W/ LEMON & OLIVE OIL 1 GLASS RED WINE FROZEN BERRIES W/ LOW-FAT WHIPPED CREAM

WEDNESDAY	
BREAKFAST	2 EGG OMELET W/ LOW-FAT CHEDDAR CHEESE 1 SLICE WHOLE GRAIN TOAST 8 OZ POMEGRANATE JUICE GREEN TEA OR BLACK COFFEE
LUNCH	LARGE GARDEN SALAD W/ BABY SPINACH, TOMATO, BROC-COLI, AVOCADO, ALMOND SLIVERS EXTRA-VIRGIN OLIVE OIL AND VINEGAR DRESSING BROTH-BASED SOUP
DINNER	6 OZ GRILLED OR BAKED ORGANIC CHICKEN 8 OZ LONG GRAIN WILD RICE SMALL GARDEN SALAD 1 GLASS RED WINE GREEN TEA OR BLACK COFFEE 4 OZ DARK CHOCOLATE

THURSDAY	
BREAKFAST	1 CUP HIGH-FIBER LOW-SUGAR BREAKFAST CEREAL 1 CUP SOY MILK WHEY PROTEIN SHAKE 8 OZ 100% ORANGE JUICE GREEN TEA OR BLACK COFFEE
LUNCH	GARDENBURGER W/ AVOCADO & LOW-FAT SOUR CREAM 2 SLICES WHOLE GRAIN BREAD 1 CUP FRESH STRAWBERRIES 8 OZ BLACK BEAN SOUP
DINNER	WHOLE GRAIN PASTA W/ GARLIC, TOMATO, & EXTRA VIRGIN OLIVE OIL GARDEN SALAD W/ BABY SPINACH, BROCCOLI, TOMATO, AVOCADO, CHICK PEAS AND WALNUTS 1 GLASS RED WINE GREEN TEA OR BLACK COFFEE FRESH BLUEBERRIES W/ LIGHT WHIPPED CREAM

FRIDAY	
BREAKFAST	2 CUPS OATMEAL 1 CUP FRESH BLUEBERRIES 4 EGG WHITES POMEGRANATE JUICE GREEN TEA OR BLACK COFFEE
LUNCH	LARGE GARDEN SALAD W/ BABY SPINACH, TOMATO, BROCCOLI, AVOCADO, ALMOND SLIVERS EXTRA-VIRGIN OLIVE OIL AND VINEGAR DRESSING
DINNER	TURKEY CHILI (SELECT EXTRA LEAN TURKEY) WHOLE GRAIN ROLL 1 GLASS RED WINE GREEN TEA OR BLACK COFFEE 4 OZ DARK CHOCOLATE

SATURDAY	
BREAKFAST	1 CUP LOW-FAT ORGANIC YOGURT 1 CUP MIXED BERRIES SOY PROTEIN SHAKE W/ GROUND FLAX SEED ADDED 8 OZ LOW-SODIUM V8 JUICE GREEN TEA OR BLACK COFFEE
LUNCH	1-2 SLICES WHOLE WHEAT VEGETABLE PIZZA MADE W/ LOW-FAT CHEESE
DINNER	MEAL OF CHOICE - ENJOY!

SUNDAY	
BREAKFAST	MEAL OF CHOICE - ENJOY!
LUNCH	MEAL OF CHOICE - ENJOY!
DINNER	MEAL OF CHOICE - ENJOY!

SNACKS (BETWEEN MEALS)

HANDFUL OF ALMONDS OR WALNUTS
SLICED APPLE W/ PEANUT BUTTER
LOW-CARB PROTEIN SHAKE (SEE BELOW)
LOW-CARB PROTEIN BAR
FLAT BREAD W/ HUMMUS
RAW VEGETABLE STICKS W/ HUMMUS
BANANA
BAKED TORTILLA CHIPS W/ SALSA
LIGHT MICROWAVE POPCORN
UNSALTED PRETZELS
FLAVORED RICE CAKES
STRAWBERRIES W/ FAT-FREE HALF & HALF
LOW-FAT ORGANIC YOGURT W/ BERRIES
LOW-FAT COTTAGE CHEESE W/ FRESH FRUIT
100% PURE APPLE SAUCE
LOW-FAT STRING CHEESE
SLICED AVOCADO OR TOMATO
BAKED TORTILLA CHIPS W/ GUACAMOLE
DRIED FRUIT OR TRAIL MIX

PROTEIN SHAKE RECIPE

---

2 Scoops Whey or Soy Protein
2 Tbsp Ground Flaxseed
1/2 Cup Frozen Blueberries
8 OZ Skim Milk or Soy Milk

APPENDIX B

Impotence Myths and Facts

Myth: ED is an inevitable part of aging.
Fact: The causes of ED tend to go along with the aging process, such as vascular disease and high blood pressure. Also, it may take decades for a lifestyle choice, such as lack of exercise, to start kicking in adverse effects upon the penis.

Myth: Young men do not experience impotence.
Fact: This is completely false. In fact, it is said that one out of 10 men over the age of 21 are bound to encounter erectile dysfunction. The causes of these cases are more likely due to the mental health of the patient rather than his physical well-being.

Myth: Tight underwear can cause ED.
Fact: There is no proof to support this misconception.

Myth: Bicycling may be a cause of ED.
Fact: The only time ED may result from riding a bike is when it's done for long distances, without breaks, and using certain types of seats. This in no way means you should give up your long mountain bike excursions.

Myth: ED must mean a man is no longer interested in sex.
Fact: The inability to get or sustain an erection has nothing to do with being aroused by one's partner. A man with impotence can still ejaculate sperm.

Myth: My partner will leave me once I become impotent.
Fact: Though erectile dysfunctions may have a negative effect on couples, there are many treatments available now to address this problem. Reports have shown that couples who have undergone these treatments have experienced a great improvement in the quality of their relationships.

Myth: "Real men" don't experience impotence.
Fact: ALL men over the age of 30 experience impotence at least once in their lifetime. It's estimated that over 150 million men worldwide have impotence; in fact, reports suggest this figure could be as high as 300 million or more. Estimating the numbers is difficult because fewer than 2 men in 10 seek treatment for impotence problems.

Myth: Impotence is "all in the mind."
Fact: Less than 20% of impotence cases have a primary psychological cause. The majority of men with impotence have an underlying physical condition such as diabetes, heart disease, high blood pressure or prostate cancer. Stress, anxiety and loss of self-esteem are often secondary psychological factors that occur if the impotence remains undiagnosed and untreated.

Myth: Impotence is a man's problem
Fact: Both partners in a relationship can experience problems when impotence goes untreated. Often, failure to communicate and denial of the problem lead to depression, anxiety, and lack of self-esteem for both partners. A tendency to avoid sexual contact can often leave the partner feeling unloved, unattractive and unwanted.

Myth: I only need to speak with my doctor about impotence if I am sexually active.
Fact: Impotence can be an early warning sign of cardiovascular disease, the number one cause of death in the U.S. You should always inform your doctor of any sudden changes in your ability to achieve or maintain an erection, so that he or she may rule out the possibility of illness or disease.

ADDENDUM

For those of you who are just not sure if you even have a problem, consider this device from www.FastSize.com. It is called the Fastsize Erectile Quality Meter (EQM). The difficulty with determining if an erection is a good one is that as men we have no standard to measure against. It is quite embarrassing to even think about asking your best buddy, "Hey how hard do you get?" or "Hey can you break a brick with that thing?" Standing at attention is a happy thing to see, but how do you know if your erection can actually perform for you? The EQM is designed to test this aspect of your erection. It is a handheld device, battery-powered, that is held against the tip of your erect penis and the pressure exerted on the testing surface will produce an electric current in the device. This will turn on a tiny lightbulb and the color of the light will tell you your axial strength (tip to base, not side to side). Blue color is the best and tells you that you have nothing to worry about-yet. Remember that an ounce of prevention is worth a pound of cure, so take care now to make a difference in your diet and exercise to avoid this problem.

www.ingramcontent.com/pod-product-compliance
Lightning Source LLC
Chambersburg PA
CBHW020336290526
45785CB00005B/2048